REFORMING
HEALTHCARE

Reforming Healthcare

How to Fix the System without the Destruction of the American Way

Thomas J. Scurlock, III

To order additional copies of this book, contact:
Xlibris
844-714-8691
www.Xlibris.com
Orders@Xlibris.com
747174

CONTENTS

Part II   The Philosophy of Designing a Health Care System

FOREWORD

As a young physician struggling through years of study, staying up late on call and sacrificing time to my clients, I thrived on the idea that I was making a difference. Learning about the healing arts was a very special blessing that few had the opportunity to experience. Every day I rejoiced in the fact that I had a chance to transform another person's life. All I had to do was show up. I did not have to wait for Thanksgiving or Christmas to give gifts or to spend time with a suffering soul. All I had to do was go to work. During those eight (rarely) to sixteen hour days I was given the privilege of helping to heal others.

A change gradually started. It was imperceptible at first, hardly noticeable and easily explained away. After twenty years it became a battle to spend more than fifteen minutes with anyone who came into my office, including colleagues seeking consultation. All the while medical professionals knew that we were being given less and less time to hear our patients concerns, to examine them properly or to render a sound diagnosis. Even worse, we frequently failed at initiating the necessary treatment plan by not properly explaining it to the patient. Never mind answering their questions or ministering to their needs, just write the prescription and hope the side effects are few! Physician extenders were added to the desperate effort to give proper care, but then they too were connived into carrying huge caseloads of people who they rarely, if ever got to know. The medical and nursing associations folded. The co-pays appeared and kept climbing.

No matter what anyone says of Hillary Clinton, I will never forget her valiant effort as First Lady, to change the course of America's out of control health costs. How can we be the greatest country in the world and not be able to address this problem? How can we be the richest nation on earth and not provide for the health of our citizens? I sometimes wonder, how many have died because all those years ago, we chose profit over compassion?

I have been waiting for an answer. I have even prayed for an answer. So I knew that an answer was out there and I knew it would eventually emerge. I won't pretend to understand all of the economic principles outlined in this rescue plan. I will simply say, it can be done. We can provide sound health and life preserving care to all Americans. There will still be enough money for those who think profit is more important...just not as much.

Gina Orton, M.D.

Reform Health Care?

There is no worse tyranny than to force a man to pay for what he does not want merely because you think it would be good for him.

—Robert A. Heinlein, *The Moon Is a Harsh Mistress*

Why is it that 6.5 million people decided to pay a fine rather than sign up for the Affordable Care Act (ACA)? Maybe the bigger question is, Why did only 12.2 million people decide to sign up for the ACA when the program was supposed to serve the needs of the 50 million or so people without health care in the United States? Some people would say that it was political, and some people may say that the Affordable Care Act was not affordable. If the answer is political, will the country ever unite enough to have a health care plan that would serve the needs of all the people and do it effectively, efficiently, and inexpensively? If the answer is that health care is ultimately too expensive for some to acquire or too expensive for the government to provide, will some people ultimately accept that not everyone will have health care? One thing that we all know is that if the health care system in the United States were perfect and everyone could afford coverage, nobody would be making a fuss, and the world would look at the United States and would implement our system instead of us having arguments over how to fix health care in the country.

The health care system in the United States is wasteful, inefficient, and at the same time, incredible. Before the Patient Protection and Affordable Care Act, 264 million people out of the 319 million people in the country or about 84% in the country had some sort of health insurance. Insurance companies made a profit, pharmaceutical companies made a profit, health care providers made a profit, advances were being made in curing illnesses, and people were reasonably healthy. So why would anyone complain about a system like that? The simple answer is 16% does not have coverage.

There are four major reasons that people are dissatisfied with the health care system in the United States follows: the working poor cannot afford coverage, the sick cannot afford coverage, the old go broke with a long-term illness, and some people believe that there are better health care systems available around the world. Because of these four issues and the knowledge that the United States has the highest cost of health care in the world, there are people who want to reform the health care system. The belief that some hold is that health care is a right, and everyone in the country should have access to some basic form of health care. The belief that health care is a right is backed up by the World Health Organization.

The argument as to whether health care is a right has led to a split in the country. There are two factions that are making the right statements or maybe asking the right questions. The first faction is asking the question, "Why can't we provide health care for everyone since this country is the most prosperous country in the world?" The second faction is asking two questions: "How much is it going to cost?" and "How are we going to pay for it?"

The purpose of this project is to develop a philosophy for building a comprehensive health care system that will serve 100% of the population of the United States for about half of the current cost and then build it. The reason this needs to happen is because the country is at a proverbial fork in the road when it comes to health care. The biggest political issues of today are health care, health care, and how to pay for health care. This project will look at the health care industry and the government and public sentiment through the lens of economics and finance to determine how the systems work currently and how they can be fixed.

That being said, there will be two parts to this project. The first part will focus on how health care works both in the United States and in other countries. The second part of the project will be focused on building a philosophy and developing the most efficient and effective system for running health care in the United States.

THE STATE OF HEALTH CARE IN THE UNITED STATES

Where are we now in the United States when it comes to health care? It is 2020, there is about to be an election, and the country has just completed about six years of the ACA. Before the ACA was passed in 2010, there were about 319 million people in the country and between Medicare, Medicaid, and private insurance, 264 million people were covered with some form of payment for health care. That means that give or take, 55 million people did not have a method to pay for health care other than cash. As of 2018, there are about 330 million people in this country and 91.2% of the country is covered by some form of health care. About 23 million people gained coverage due to the ACA. The 23 million is comprised of about 12 million that gained coverage via the expansion of Medicaid and about 11 million who gained coverage through ACA marketplaces. For the purposes of clarity, because of the effects of the ACA, some statistics will be quoted in before-ACA numbers, and some will be quoted in 2018 numbers. The reason is that the effect of the ACA is clear and will serve as an example as to the way that any health care system can affect the lives and finances of the country's citizens.

There is a clarity in numbers that will show exactly why people are upset with the health care system in the United States. To start with, before the ACA took effect in 2014, health insurance cost, on average, $5,900 per person per year. By the end of 2017, this cost had increased to about $6,700 per person per year. This means that the cost of health insurance rose by 14% in about three years. The hurting part of this equation is that when the ACA was proposed, the promise was that the cost of health care for the average family would decrease by $2,500. The cost actually increased by more than $250 per year. In 2018, the average cost of health insurance for a family was $19,600 and $6,900 for an individual. The median household income was about $56,000. This means that 35% of household income would go to cover the average family if not for company-sponsored plans.

Average Health Insurance Premium			
Year	Per capita	individual	family
2009	$ 3,131.00	$ 4,824.00	$ 13,375.00
2010	$ 8,394.00	$ 5,049.00	$ 13,770.00
2011	$ 3,625.00	$ 5,429.00	$ 15,073.00
2012	$ 8,908.00	$ 5,615.00	$ 15,745.00
2013	$ 9,113.00	$ 5,884.00	$ 16,351.00
2014	$ 9,518.00	$ 6,025.00	$ 16,834.00
2015	$ 9,995.00	$ 6,251.00	$ 17,545.00
2016	$ 10,379.00	$ 6,435.00	$ 18,142.00
2017	$ 10,742.00	$ 6,690.00	$ 18,764.00
2018	$ 11,172.00	$ 6,896.00	$ 19,616.00

The individual and family date came from Kaiser Family foundation. www. kff.org and the per capita data https://www.statista.com/statistics/184955/ us-national-health-expenditures-per-capita-since-1960/

The cost of health insurance has led to Senator Bernie Sanders proposing "Medicare for All." This proposal would eliminate health insurance companies and install a government-run health care system. On the other side of this equation, the Republicans are proposing Health Savings Accounts to offset the cost of health care. All of this is because the United States spends $450 billion per year in prescription drugs (https://www.reuters.com/article/ us-usa-drugspending-quintilesims-idUSKBN1800BU) and more than $250 billion to combat type 2 diabetes (https://www.cdc.gov/chronicdisease/ resources/publications/aag/diabetes.htm). It is interesting to note that type 2 diabetes accounts for almost 10% of all health care costs before the ACA and continues to increase in cost to the health care system. Type 2 diabetes is a chronic illness, and chronic illnesses are the number one reason that health care costs are so high in the United States.

According to the Centers for Disease Control, a chronic disease is a disease lasting three months or longer. About 40 million Americans are limited in their usual activities due to one or more chronic health conditions (https://www.cdc.gov/nchs/data/series/sr_10/sr10_259.pdf). Generally incurable and ongoing, chronic diseases affect approximately 133 million Americans, representing more than 40% of the total population of this country (https://www.cdc.gov/chronicdisease/pdf/2009-Power-of-Prevention.pdf). By 2020, that number is projected to grow to an estimated 157 million, with 81 million having multiple conditions (https://www.thelancet.com/journals/lancet/article/PIIS0140-6736(09)60048-9/fulltext).

Ninety percent of the nation's $3.3 trillion in annual health care expenditures are for people with chronic or mental health conditions (https://www.cdc.gov/chronicdisease/about/costs/index.htm). That means that cancer, diabetes, hypertension, stroke, heart disease, pulmonary conditions, Alzheimer's disease, tooth decay, arthritis, and mental illness are the drivers behind 90% of all health care costs in this country. Before the ACA, 47% of people with a chronic illness did not have a payment method for health care other than cash.

One of the solutions that continues to be suggested is to provide preventative care, and that will stop people from getting chronic illnesses. If that worked, then why do 81 million people in this country have more than one chronic illness? There must be a way to slow the growth of chronic illnesses so that the costs do not overwhelm the health care system. Maybe the real problem is lifestyle. If everyone who was at risk for type 2 diabetes would eat healthy and exercise, the cost of health care could be cut, and everyone would be able to afford at least basic care.

Most people are aware that 31% of all medical expenses a person will incur are in the last year of their lives. This is the reason that is given for the high cost of Medicare. This could be true. But there is another statistic that tells us that 1% of the population incurs 20% of the health care costs. That means that over 3 million people spent more than $90,000 per year in health care. On the flip side of that equation, about 50% spent less than $250 per year (https://www.thebalance.com/healthcare-costs-3306068). The easy fix is to euthanize the 3 million, and health care costs would be low enough for everyone to afford them. That is not an option.

Some people are upset because of the cost of prescription drugs. The cost of a prescription dose of a drug for Crohn's disease could be as high as

$2,900 (https://www.drugs.com/price-guide/humira). That is a high price to pay. The worldwide revenue for pharmaceutical companies is over $1.05 trillion with profits of 21%. $515 billion of that revenue comes from the United States and Canada. These two countries make up 7% of the world population (https://www.fool.com/investing/2016/07/31/12-big-pharma-stats-that-will-blow-you-away.aspx). Maybe the drug companies should be made to operate on a nonprofit basis. That would save the world $200 billion. The question is would that slow or stop that quest for new drugs?

There are thousands of questions to ask about health care. The answers to some of the questions are simple, and some are complicated. Before answering complicated questions or any other questions, it is essential to understand that when politics is brought into the discussion, the most relevant issues will be addressed. Before these issues are addressed and the first real complicated question are posed, it is important to understand the current system.

How Does the United States Compare to the World?

In the United States when people get sick or hurt, they go to a doctor, hospital, or other type of health care facility (health care provider). The person receives treatment, and the health care provider expects payment for their services. This seems simple. It gets more complicated if the person in need of care has cancer or a chronic illness. In these cases, the treatment could cost more than the person has available or may earn in a lifetime. What has happened is that the government and private industry have decided to allow these people to transfer their risk of illness or injury for a fee. This fee has gotten higher than some people can afford, which leaves them without health care coverage and without the ability to pay out of pocket for said care. This is a very simplified explanation that doesn't address insurance companies, Medicaid, Medicare, or the Patient Protection and Affordable Care Act (ACA). The details of how the health care system works in the United States will be discussed later, but now there is a basis to answer a few complicated questions.

How does the United States health care system compare to the universal health care systems in the world? Before the ACA, there were about 84% of people in the United States covered by some type of health coverage. The truth of the matter is none of the universal health care systems in the world hit 100% coverage of 100% of their citizens. There is always a mix of coverage and percentages of public coverage and private insurance. For example, in France, it is mandatory that everyone have insurance. However, not everything is covered, and 92% of the French have private insurance. In Germany, only 88% of the population is covered by the state:

"approximately 31 percent of the German population purchase private supplemental insurance and close to 11 percent of citizens have signed full private health insurance since their income is high enough to exempt them from statutory insurance requirements" (http://www.deloitte.com/assets/Dcom-UnitedStates/Local%20Assets/Documents/US_CHS_2011ConsumerSurveyGlobal_062111.pdf). Mexico only covers about 85% of their population, and Canada covers everyone. However, there is a need for 75% of the population to carry private insurance (Deloitte.com).

The private auditing firm Deloitte did a survey in 2011 and found that in the countries with health care systems in Europe, the percentage of people who would rate their country's health care at an *A* or *B* ranged from about 40 to 50%, and in the United States, 22% would rate the system an *A* or *B*. Yes, the European systems are grouped together. The question is, if a single payer system is so good then, why is the satisfaction rate so low? You would think that people would be happier, maybe 75% satisfied. However, what sticks out is only 22% of those surveyed in the United States would give the health care system a grade of *A* or *B*. What is interesting about the study is that the people surveyed in the United States view themselves as the healthiest in the world.

The real problem with the health care system in the United States is the cost. There are a few people, about 130 million, who have preexisting conditions that insurance companies will not cover or charge higher prices to cover their risk, so some of those people are unable to shift the risk of illness. Moreover, the biggest reason that people file for bankruptcy is medical bills: 66.5% of all bankruptcies are caused by medical bills (https://www.nasdaq.com/articles/medical-bankruptcy-is-killing-the-american-middle-class-2019-02-14). These reasons have led to an outcry to reform the system. There have been movies like *Sicko* that bring awareness to the issues of the health care system in the United States and compare it to a few health care systems around the world. Since 1947, The World Health Organization has been calling for all countries to provide universal health care and advocating for health care as a right. What this led to is mass dissatisfaction with the system and a call for reform. What most people don't realize is that the problems and solutions to health care are rooted in two issues, risk and cost.

The Patient Protection and Affordable Care Act

Over the past fifty years or so, health care has been changing to meet demands and to keep up with technology. Insurance has changed, and so have government programs. As these programs change and people become aware of how other countries are handling the cost of health care, attitudes change toward the system in the United States. Some people look at the systems that are in place in the UK and Canada and believe that since those countries have a payment mechanism for 100% of their citizens, the systems are superior to ours. Because of this, people have started believing that health care is a right, and in a country as prosperous as the United States, the government should be able to provide health care for everyone. This issue has led to the development and the implementation of the Patient Protection and Affordable Care Act.

The Patient Protection and Affordable Care Act, or Obamacare as it is referred to, is a system that aims to cover about 20 million of the 50 million people not covered by some type of health care payment system. Obamacare (the ACA) includes a patient bill of rights and encourages individuals and companies to participate. This is the first step that the government has provided to bridge the gap in coverage for the 16% without some sort of health care coverage. This bill of rights is the first step toward the goals of the World Health Organization to provide universal health care for everyone.

Patient's Bill of Rights

(https://www.whitehouse.gov/files/documents/
healthcare-fact-sheets/patients-bill-rights.pdf)

- Ban on Discriminating Against Kids with Pre-Existing Conditions

Before reform, tens of the thousands of families have been denied insurance each year for their children because of an illness or condition. With the Patient's Bill of Rights, plans cannot discriminate against kids with preexisting conditions. In 2014, no one seeking coverage can be discriminated against because of a preexisting condition.

- Ban on Insurance Companies Dropping Coverage

Before reform, insurance companies could cancel your coverage when you were sick and needed it most because of a simple mistake on your application. With the Patient's Bill of Rights, insurance companies are banned from cutting off your coverage due to an unintentional mistake on your application.

- Ban on Insurance Companies Limiting Coverage

Before reform, cancer patients and individuals suffering from other serious and chronic diseases were often forced to limit or go without treatment because of an insurer's lifetime limit on their coverage. With the Patient's Bill of Rights, insurance companies can no longer put a lifetime limit on the amount of coverage so families can live with the security of knowing that their coverage will be there when they need it most. The use of annual limits was restricted and banned completely in 2014.

- Ban on Insurance Companies Limiting Choice of Doctors

Before reform, insurance companies could decide which doctor you could go to. With the Patient's Bill of Rights, if you purchase or join a new plan, you have the right to choose your own doctor in your insurer network.

- Ban on Insurance Companies Restricting Emergency Room Care

Before reform, insurance companies could limit which emergency room you could go to or charge you more if you went out of network. With the Patient's Bill of Rights, if you purchase or join a new plan, those plans are banned from charging more for emergency services obtained out of network.

- Guarantee You a Right to Appeal

Before reform, when insurers denied you coverage or restricted your treatment, you were left with few options to repeal. With the Patient's Bill of Rights, if you purchase or join a new policy, you will be guaranteed the right to appeal insurance company decisions to an independent third party.

- Covering Young Adults on Parents' Plan

With the Patient's Bill of Rights, young adults will be allowed to remain on their parents' plan until their twenty-sixth birthday unless they are offered coverage at work. Up to 2.4 million young adults could gain affordable coverage through this provision of the new law.

- Covering Preventive Care with No Cost

With the Patient's Bill of Rights, if you join or purchase a new plan, you will receive recommended preventive care with no out-of-pocket cost. Services like mammograms, colonoscopies, immunizations, prenatal and new-baby care will be covered, and insurance companies will be prohibited from charging deductibles, copayments, or coinsurance.

Without judgments on whether health care is a right, there are several questions that arise from the implementation of the Patient Protection and Affordable Care Act (ACA). Why didn't the United States pass and implement a government-sponsored single-payer health care system like they have in Canada or the UK? What will be the effect of the ACA on the current health care system? What will happen to Medicare and Medicaid? How much will the ACA ultimately cost? How will the government pay for the new health care system? There are other questions, but we have a start.

The History of Health Insurance

Before Germany implemented a state-run health care system in the 1880s, there was no insurance to pay for health care worldwide. In the United States, as early as the 1860s, a few companies started selling accident insurance. Later in the 1920s, a few hospitals started offering plans to people in the community to pay for procedures that would be too costly to handle all at once. This grew into an industry for those who could afford to pay, and health insurance was born.

As things evolved, health insurance was offered by employers as a benefit of employment. The industry and the country continued to evolve, and eventually, the government got into the business of providing what was called Medicare for the elderly that the insurance companies wouldn't cover. More evolution occurred, and the government gave the poor Medicaid.

A couple of years ago, there was a call for coverage for everyone, so now we have the ACA. In other words, about 50 million people are covered by Medicare, about 70 million people are covered by Medicaid, about 150 million people are covered by private insurance, and about 50 million people are uninsured. In 2014, when the ACA went into effect, about 40 million were uninsured, and about 11 million were covered under the ACA. The other numbers remained about the same. (The numbers are rounded to make it easy to follow.)

Everyone is not covered, and we have five types of health care coverage, which range from no coverage to private insurance to government-sponsored coverage. (Because of the nature of the ACA changing the coverage parameters of insurance, the cost of insurance will be quoted based on pre-ACA figures. Pre-ACA risk was calculated differently, which changed the cost of coverage. There will be times when post-ACA numbers will be quoted for the purpose of current comparisons.)

Why the ACA?

Earlier, there were some questions about the move to the ACA. The first was why didn't the United States implement a single-payer system instead or the ACA? That is a hard question to answer. It has several answers. First, the perception of universal health care or socialized medicine carries the perception of socialism to some Americans. This goes against the beliefs of some Americans, and a full rollout of a universal health care system would not have passed the House and Senate to be written into law. Second, some requirements of a single-payer system may violate the Constitution. Third, the private health care providers may have lobbied against the system, and a single-payer system would eliminate some of them. Fourth, there is the cost or perceived cost of a universal health care system. The reasons go on and on, but the real argument can be boiled down to one phrase: some people think it is un-American.

What will be the effect of the ACA on the current health care system? As of 2017, there were about 11 million people enrolled in the ACA, 12 million that have been added to Medicaid, 6.5 million had elected to pay the penalty and declined insurance, and the rest of the people were just not covered. That means that more people have declined the ACA than elected to utilize health care through the ACA. The cost per person per year of private health insurance has climbed from about $5,400 in 2011 to more than $6,700 in 2017. The cost of Medicaid has been mostly unchanged during this period. In the long term, there must be changes, or not just the ACA will fail but the entire health care industry will have difficulty as well. Ultimately, the government will have to double down and pay to save the ACA, or the system will have to be scrapped and a new system will have to be put in place.

What will happen to Medicare and Medicaid? Under the current system, nothing will happen to Medicare and Medicaid. Former President Barack Obama has stated that there is more than 30% fraud and waste in the systems, but to this point, there has been no effort to fix the system. To be realistic, Medicare will probably have a larger role in health care, eventually becoming the system that will be used for all of health care. There is a push for Medicare for everyone.

How much will the ACA cost? This is the hardest question in the world to answer. There has been over $1 trillion spent on the ACA before it was implemented, and the CBO estimates a cost of about $250 billion per year to serve 20 million people. The reality, as of the end of 2017, is that the ACA is directly serving about 11 million people. The Republicans promised to get rid of it, and so far, Congress has voted to defund the rebates to insurance companies. Currently, the ACA is like Schrodinger's cat—it is both alive and dead.

Universal Health Care

One of the most important parts of building a new health care system is to understand what is already out there, how they work, and the philosophies of the systems. Perhaps the most important influence on health care around the world came in 1948 when the World Health Organization declared health care to be a right and that all countries should provide universal health care for all of their citizens. About the same time in Europe, the UK instituted their first state-run health care system, and over the next fifty years, "universal" health care systems have been popping up in various countries around the world.

It seems that the rest of the world has bought into the ideas of the World Health Organization, but not the United States of America. The World Health Organization stated that,

> The goal of universal health coverage is to ensure that all people obtain the health services they need without suffering financial hardship when paying for them.

> For a community or country to achieve universal health coverage, several factors must be in place, including:

> 1. A strong, efficient, well-run health system that meets priority health needs through people-centered integrated care (including services for HIV, tuberculosis, malaria, non-communicable diseases, maternal and child health) by:
>   ○ informing and encouraging people to stay healthy and prevent illness;
>   ○ detecting health conditions early;

- ○ having the capacity to treat disease; and
- ○ Helping patients with rehabilitation.

2. Affordability – a system for financing health services so people do not suffer financial hardship when using them. This can be achieved in a variety of ways.

3. Access to essential medicines and technologies to diagnose and treat medical problems.

4. A sufficient capacity of well-trained, motivated health workers to provide the services to meet patients' needs based on the best available evidence.

It also requires recognition of the critical role played by all sectors in assuring human health, including transport, education and urban planning.

Universal health coverage has a direct impact on a population's health. Access to health services enables people to be more productive and active contributors to their families and communities. It also ensures that children can go to school and learn. At the same time, financial risk protection prevents people from being pushed into poverty when they have to pay for health services out of their own pockets. Universal health coverage is thus a critical component of sustainable development and poverty reduction, and a key element of any effort to reduce social inequities. Universal coverage is the hallmark of a government's commitment to improve the wellbeing of all its citizens.

Universal coverage is firmly based on the WHO constitution of 1948 declaring health a fundamental human right and on the Health for All agenda set by the Alma-Ata declaration in 1978. Equity is paramount. This means that countries need to track progress not just across the national population but within different groups (e.g. by income level, sex, age, place of residence, migrant status and ethnic origin).

This definition is in line with the arguments that the proponents of a universal health care system espouse. Furthermore, it goes on to state that health care is a "fundamental human right." This is the foundation for the plan that will arise for the people of the United States. Keep each of the tenets of the World Health Organization in mind as we move on.

RISK AND COST

There are risks and costs to action. But they are far less than the long-range risks of comfortable inaction.

—John F. Kennedy

Michael Milken

In the 1980s, there was an investment banker named Michael Milken. He worked for a company named Drexel Burnham Lambert. Mr. Milken is famous for developing a market for high-yield bonds, also known as junk bonds. Mr. Milken discovered that there were several companies that needed financing that had less-than-desirable credit. The risk of default on debt financing for these companies was high. Some of those companies were smaller local or regional savings banks. The problem was that he would have to do two things: convince the companies that they could get financing despite their credit rating and convince investors that the bonds that he issued to finance the companies would yield higher returns for their portfolio.

Mr. Milken understood the risk that he was taking and the potential gains that could prove very helpful to everyone involved in his venture. To convince investors to purchase the investment in high-yield bonds, he told them that the bonds carried much higher interest rates than investment grade bonds. In some cases, bond yields could be over 20%. In other words, a risk-averse investor will need a higher yield to offset the risk in an investment. This is a simple concept explained by risk-free rate. Essentially, risk-free rate is the interest rate that carries no risk. In general, it is pegged to the ten-year U.S. Treasury note. This rate over the past fifty years or so is about 4.3%. As the risk in an investment increases, the corresponding yield of the investment must rise.

The biggest issues with junk bonds are that sometimes the interest was so high or the amount issued exceeded what the issuer could pay. This would cause the issuer to refinance the bond to pay the investors. This was great for Mr. Milken because he was standing ready to handle the business.

The problems for Mr. Milken began in about 1986 when arbitrageur Ivan Boesky was indicted and implicated Mr. Milken in wrongdoing. This was the beginning of the end for the junk bond industry in the 1980s. Without Mr. Milken to refinance the bonds, some of the banks that had been financed by Drexel Burnham Lambert began to collapse. This led to the stock market crash in 1987 and what is called the savings and loan crises.

RISK

When Michael Milken sold bonds for his clients, because the risk of the bonds was high, the cost to the issuer was high, up to about 20% interest. Risk is always a driver of cost. As the risk increases, the cost increases. If the risk involved with a product or service grows, the cost of the product can rise beyond the ability of the consumer to purchase the product. Furthermore, the greater the risk, the higher the chances of default. This is the exact situation with health care.

"A 1985 federal law requires emergency departments to stabilize and treat anyone entering their doors, regardless of their ability to pay. While hospitals average 7% profit margins, uncompensated care costs can be more than 5% of revenue. The year the Affordable Care Act passed, hospitals provided about $40 billion in 'uncompensated care'—that is, care they were not paid for. That was nearly 6% of their total 2010 expenses" (https://www.usatoday.com/story/news/politics/2017/07/03/who-pays-when-someone-without-insurance-shows-up-er/445756001/).

In this situation, the hospitals have payment risk. Payment risk means that as long as there are people without some method of payment for health care other than cash, the provider of the service will run the risk of nonpayment. To offset this risk, hospitals must raise prices for the services provided. This goes on throughout the entire health care system in the United States. It is one of the reasons that the ACA wanted everyone on one system, because in that situation, there would be little to no payment risk.

The ACA changed the way that risk was assessed in the United States. Before the ACA, 47% of those with chronic illnesses couldn't obtain insurance or were turned down for insurance. The reason was adverse selection. This created an issue for the health insurance companies in the United States. How do they address risk? The real problems with health care in the United States are not really the working poor not being able to afford coverage, the sick not being able to afford coverage, the old going broke with a long-term illness, and some people believing that there are better health care systems available around the world. The real reasons that people are dissatisfied are risk and cost. They just don't know that is the reason. Risk and cost are the reasons that our system costs more than systems around the world. The way we manage risk and costs determines who gets the best coverage and the cost of that coverage. The insurance companies in this country in some cases will cover everything if the payment is enough for the coverage, whereas in other countries in the world, they manage risk and costs much differently than we do here.

France was considered the top-rated health care system in the world in 2000, yet they don't cover all chronic illnesses. In France, even though they may cover 100% of the people, most of them, about 92%, have private insurance to cover what is not covered by the government. Japan is currently considered the top-rated system in the world. In Japan, the people are required to have insurance to subsidize the government plan and must pay 30% coinsurance (the elderly have different percentages to pay based on age).

The government programs Medicare, Medicaid, and the Patient Protection and Affordable Care Act (ACA) have differing views. Currently the government is willing to take on some unlimited risk and some limited risk; there is no expectation of profit. The limited risk is because Medicare has a set schedule of fixed payments and time limitations. The unlimited risk is because Medicaid and the ACA either capped the out-of-pocket expenses of the individual or the individual doesn't have payment responsibility. However, private insurance is willing to take risks that are below the threshold of profit. This creates another problem: private insurance companies are not willing to take on those who are ill before applying for coverage, or the coverage may be so costly that the individual cannot afford that expense. In this case, the individual is left responsible for the entire cost of treatment. When this happens, there may be bankruptcy because of cost of treatment or loss of life because of delays or denial of service.

Because of the ACA, there is a perception that everyone will be covered by insurance or some payment method for health care. This is not the case all the time. Since 2014, the cost of insurance, even the ACA plans, has grown faster than the rate of inflation. In some cases, rates have doubled or tripled for some people. There are several reasons for this increase. One of which is the Patient's Bill of Rights. Before, the ACA insurance companies could exclude some people based on the risk to the pool of their customers. This is called adverse selection. In France, this system is used. France covers about thirty chronic illnesses; however, they do not cover everything. France mandates that their citizens carry insurance that cover the chronic illnesses that the country doesn't cover. France also doesn't pay 100% of the cost of an illness or injury. They allow the insurance companies to cover that issue. This is one of the ways that a country manages risk. This is also the way the insurance companies used to handle risk.

Risk is nothing more than the potential of loss or gain based on activity or inactivity. In health care, there is risk for the individual, the insurance provider, the government, and the health care provider. These risks determine costs and behavior. The individual is faced with a few decisions at various times in his life based on risk. Some people view their risk of illness as low and choose not to carry some form of health care coverage. This can be because the cost of coverage is more than the cost of the service required. It is a simple equation: If a person doesn't believe that he will be sick or have a catastrophic health event during the year, he figures the cost of going to the doctor a few times of the year and compares it to the cost of coverage for the year. If he feels the cost of coverage exceeds the cost of service, the decision is an easy one—save the difference and do not pay for coverage.

Conversely, there are some people who think they have a higher risk of illness and choose to carry some form of coverage. The equation is the same as above: the person weighs the cost of coverage versus the cost of paying for services out of pocket. There are people who, because of the limits of their income, cannot afford the cost of health care coverage, so the equation is easy for them and fortunately don't get sick. Unfortunately, there are some people who were either born with an illness or contracted some illness or injury that, because of the system, do not have the opportunity to make a decision on coverage because the risk to the coverage provider is greater than the provider is willing to take. These people must bear the cost of coverage out of pocket.

The risk factors for the latter two situations are the main reasons that there is dissatisfaction in the current health care system in the United States.

The ACA was concerned with the problem of preexisting conditions, and one of the tenets of the Patient's Bill of Rights eliminates preexisting conditions as a method of disqualification for health care coverage.

There are three major risks that a health care provider has: a risk of nonpayment from the customer, a risk of litigation, and a payment or reimbursement risk from the government or insurance company. The risk of no-payment from the individual cannot be mitigated because technically the provider cannot turn away someone in need of urgent care. These costs are projected and averaged across the projected number of patients as a cost above the actual cost of service. This total cost is passed on to the individual. This is the reason that a box of tissues may cost $90 at the hospital.

The second risk, litigation, can be mitigated by purchasing insurance. This risk is also added to the cost of service.

The third risk is a payment or reimbursement risk. Government payments are on a fixed schedule and usually are lower than private Insurance payments. There is a risk that the government or private insurance company will not pay for the service. These risks are not uniform throughout the country, and they burden some areas more than others. This makes health care costs in some areas more expensive then in others. (There are other factors and risks that may be discussed later.)

Because of the nature of government programs as a payment mechanism not designed for profit, the risk is defined as the exposure to unlimited or uncapped payments per person. The government programs Medicare, Medicaid, and the Patient Protection and Affordable Care Act (ACA) have a different view on risk. In Medicare, the government in general will pick up some costs and leave other costs to be taken care of by private insurance and the individual. There are deductibles that need to be met at timed points of service, but in general, the program boils down to an 80-20 insurance plan. This program only serves people over sixty-five years old, in end stage renal care, and those with Lou Gehrig's disease.

Medicaid is a bit different; it is a joint effort between states and the federal government for those who in general have income 133% of the poverty line or lower. For the most part, the risk is uncapped and not shared by the covered. (Some states charge copays or other types of fees.)

The ACA shares risk with those in each of the four plans; however, in the Bronze and Silver plans, the covered have their risk capped and the plan covers the remaining risk. In essence, the government plans, for the most part, shift the risk of absolute costs from the individual to the government.

Insurance companies are in business to make a profit. They have actuaries who tell them the probability of death, illness, and injury that every person they cover has and projects the cost of each illness and/or injury to the company. They are concerned with adverse selection or keeping people on their plans that will not cost them money while maximizing the revenue derived from each person. They are also concerned with excluding those who will cost them more money than they can derive in revenue. Maybe it should be said that they are concerned with limiting their exposure to sick or injured people so they will not have to pass the costs of these people to their risk pool. They view risk differently than the government or most individuals. Insurance companies limit risk by understanding the cost of illnesses and injury to the company and sharing this risk through premiums, copays, and deductibles with the people they cover.

Risk in every part of the system is dealt with differently. However, the one thing that is important about risk is other than fixed cost of providing services it is the biggest driver of health care costs in the system.

> The health care services received by uninsured individuals that they do not pay for themselves are picked up or "absorbed" by a number of parties, including:
>
> • practitioners and institutions, both public and private, that serve the uninsured at no charge or reduced charges;
> • the federal government, localities, and states that support the operation of hospitals and clinics, both through direct appropriations and implicit subsidies like the Medicare and Medicaid disproportionate share hospital payments; and
> • philanthropic donations. (https://www.ncbi.nlm.nih.gov/books/NBK221653/)

The greatest example of this fact is that about 3% of the cost of the health care system or about $90 billion is uncompensated to the system. Furthermore, about one-sixth of health care expenses are borne by people who pay out of pocket or people who have no health care coverage. This means that if this risk can be mitigated, the cost of health care can be reduced significantly.

The way that risk is mitigated in some foreign countries differs greatly from the way that risk is mitigated in the United States. Some countries in the world cover almost all the people, and the government is the payment mechanism. Because of this, the payment risk is zero. This is the major reason that the cost of these systems is less than the systems in the United States. Furthermore, in the United States, the risk is based on the individual, and the individual is charged based on his risk to the pool. In other countries, because the pool includes everyone, the risk is divided based on income, not on individual risk to the pool. This allows for everyone to share the same coverage but not at the same price. Some people do not pay at all while some pay amounts that are multiples of what they would pay if their risk was evaluated individually.

If aggregated, most of the health care systems in the world mitigate risk by sharing the cost with insurance companies. The people are required to have private insurance that would cover the cost of services that are not covered by the government. This is like insurance plans in the United States with 80-20 or 70-30 coverage. It is also similar to Medicare. In Medicare, the cost is shared by the government and, in some cases, an insurance company.

Buy.Com

In 1997, Buy.com was founded. The plan for the company was to sell computers at prices below cost on the Internet. The loses would be made up with advertisements. Initially, the company did very well in terms of sales. The first year, they had sales of over $125 million.

Buy.com did very well when it came to sales and very well when it came to raising money. The company raised money from SoftBank to offset losses and went public in 2000 with an initial public offering raising $195 million. Within one year, the losses piled up, and the stock price was below $1 per share.

In 2001, the company was delisted for failing to keep its stock price above $1. This was due to the losses that the company incurred. The founder of the company reacquired the company for about $23 million and continued to run losses. Today, the company exists as Rakuten.com as it was acquired in 2010 by the largest retailer in Japan. They have put more than $250 million into the company. The company no longer sells products below cost. They focus on a business model that offers rebates on products bought through their site.

COST

There is a lot to learn from Buy.com. The problem with selling a product or service at a loss is that at some point, the operations will have to cease. This is because if there is a product that is being sold, the company will not be able to purchase the raw materials or products needed to produce and sell their product. If it is a service, the providers of that service at some point will not be able to be paid. Either way, the company will cease to exist.

The issue of cost is the biggest issue when it comes to health care. If a person must have surgery, the hospital has costs that must be paid. The surgeon must be paid. There is a cost for blood, a cost for the nurses, a cost for the drugs, and the list of costs continue from there. What some people believe is that if the government is in control of the system, they can lower the costs of everything involved by price fixing, negotiating, and additional taxation to make up the difference. This may be true in the short run; however, over time, this may affect the entire system.

In the UK, the government controlled the health care system and employed all the doctors and health care workers. The government negotiated the prices of drugs and limited the services that were available to the people. The health care system was too costly, and in about 2012, they undertook a reorganization to change the way health care worked.

Cost is the reason that the health care system in the United States is ranked lower than some of the other systems in the world. It is not difficult to see why it cost more in the United States to secure health care. Starting at the bottom, the average salaries of a general practitioner in the United States is about $161,000. In the UK, it is about $116,000. The revenue for pharmaceutical companies in the United States is about $450 billion while worldwide revenue is about $1.02 trillion. That means that 45% of all money spent on drugs was spent in the United States. The profits for pharmaceutical companies are about 20% worldwide.

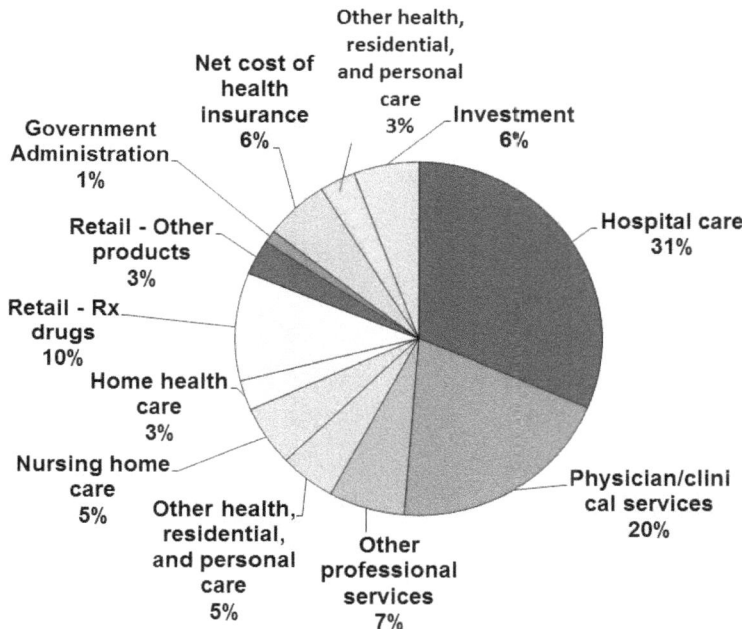

As you can see from the graph, almost $3.3 trillion in health care costs can be divided into several categories to reflect where costs occur. What the graph doesn't show is fraud and waste, risk and profits. But let's start with the basics. The graph clearly shows the percentage of dollars that are spent in each type of care. What you can clearly see is that everything has a cost. The doctors have expenses to run their offices. They need to have employees. They need to buy gauze and tongue depressors. Some doctors have EKG machines in their offices. That costs money. Malpractice costs $56 billion per year and increasing. Medical devices cost money. Surgery costs money. Building hospitals costs money. Drugs cost money. The point is that health care costs money. The fallacy that some people believe is that to reduce the cost of health care, you just nationalize it, and all the costs will go down. That is not the case.

If you took away the 3% that some doctors profit, the 5% that the insurance companies make, the profits from the tongue depressor companies, and the profits from the companies that make catheters, there will still be the need to produce these products, and there will still be the need to have skilled doctors.

Below is a chart of the cost of health care around the world.

Health Care Expenditures as Percent of GDP		Per Capita Spending ($USD)	Public Expenditure on Health, Percent of Total
Belgium	11.0%	$3,995	27.9%
Brazil	8.4%	$606	79.9%
Canada	10.4%	$4,079	70.2%
China	4.7%	$108	67.9%
France	11.4%	$3,696	77.8%
Germany	10.9%	$3,737	76.8%
Luxembourg	6.8%	$4,237	84.1%
Mexico	6.4%	$852	46.9%
Portugal	10%	$2,108	70.6%
Switzerland	11.2%	$4,627	59.1%
UK	10.1%	$3,129	82.6%
United States	17.6%	$8,086	46.5%

This chart is brilliant for what it says and for what it is implying. There is a purity in these numbers that cuts through ideology. Looking at the trend or what is recurring, the first thing that you see is in most of the countries in the chart, the percentage of GDP that is spent on health care is about 10% and the cost per capita is about $4000. But the thing that really sticks out is that the United States spends about double per capita for health care, and it consumes about 70% more of the percentage of GDP.

The question of cost is one of the biggest arguments in health care. Why does it cost twice as much for health care in the United States than it does in Europe? There can be several answers, from limitations in chronic coverage to smaller population size. Maybe the key is in the fact that we have one system to provide care and fifty-five mechanisms for payment, and all are separate (each state Medicaid system was counted as a payment mechanism). When you boil it down, the truth of the matter is bureaucracy. Waste and fraud plague the U.S. health care system. This is evident when you look at the cost of Medicaid and Medicare compared to the cost of private insurance. Medicaid has fifty states paying into a system that is matched by the federal government. Each state has different rules for their citizens and a government to administer the program, and on top of that, the federal government has their administration of a program that has unlimited exposure to cost.

What most people miss is that the median income in the United States is about $56,000 compared to about $33,000 in the UK, $6,200 in China, $33,000 in Japan, and $30,000 in France. That means that medical products manufactured in the United States are going to be more expensive than in other countries. It also means that the average salaries of doctors and nurses are going to be higher in the United States. The average salaries of the administration in doctors' offices and hospitals are going to be more expensive. This also means that it is necessary that the cost of health care products and services are going to be costlier in the United States than around the world.

As was stated before, there are about 30 million people in the United States that spend more than $90,000 per year in health care. These people are chronically ill. Chronic illness accounts for more than 90% of the cost of health care in the United States. On the flip side of the equation, about 50% of the people in the United States spend less than $250 per year in health care. It is easy to say, "We need to do something about chronic illnesses." But the truth of the matter is that there will always be those who are chronically ill and those who are healthy. That is the exact reason that insurances companies used to practice adverse selection to lower their costs.

Before the ACA, government cost about $9,000 per person covered per year (cost of Medicare and Medicaid with states contribution to Medicaid, $1 trillion/total number of people on Medicare and Medicaid 117 million = $9,000), private insurance costs about $5,900 per person per year (total revenue of health insurance industry, $860 billion/total number of people with health insurance 147 million = $5,900). The question you must ask yourself is, Why is a system where profit is required less costly than a system where no profit is required?

To go further with the cost scenario, why is it that the insurance companies can pay doctors $100–$200 per visit and pay the full price of hospital services and still be less expensive than the government plans that have a schedule that pays doctors about $30 per patient visit? Some doctors and hospitals will refuse to take people on Medicare or Medicaid for this very reason. Furthermore, because the government programs pay less per procedure, health care providers must charge more to the patients who pay full price for service. The reason is that every service or product has a cost, and that cost must be met by the provider for the good or service. If that cost is not met, the provider will go out of business.

But what happens when the government takes over the health care system and pays less than the cost of the products and services? This happens all over the world. To make health care affordable for everyone, most countries allow the people with higher incomes to subsidize those with lower incomes. Then they charge a higher tax on those who are wealthier. The government then fixes prices and salaries. In Japan, government services employ the health care staff, and nongovernment health care providers operate as nonprofit entities.

When there is no motive to make a profit and the cost of the product or service is not met, the government either fixes the prices or rations the product or service. That is why in countries like the UK and Canada some surgeries or procedures can take some time to schedule whereas in the United States currently, the waiting time for most procedures is short.

Moreover, there are other answers to why the government is costlier than private insurance. First, there is a statistic that says that 31% of all health care cost is spent in the last year of life. Medicare absorbs most of this cost because Medicare covers people over sixty-five while private insurance isn't the primary care that covers anyone over sixty-five. However, that is not the real reason. The real reason that government plans cost more than private insurance is because of bureaucracy, waste, and fraud. The cost to administer Medicare and Medicaid is between about 8% of their budget (U.S. Government Accountability Office [GAO]). To be very conservative, the cost of administration for the two government plans is about $100 billion per year. There are studies that estimate the cost of waste and fraud in Medicare and Medicaid at between 15% (GAO) and 30% (http://oversight.house.gov/wp-content/uploads/2012/04/Uncovering-Waste-Fraud-and-Abuse-in-the-Medicaid-Program-Final-3.pdf). If this is the case, that means that on the low end, 25% of all cost to run Medicare and Medicaid cover bureaucracy, fraud, and waste while 75% go to health care. That is $250 billion per year for bureaucracy, fraud, and waste.

But there has to be more reasons other than risk and cost that make some people want to change the health care system in the United States. And there are numerous problems that the United States faces both now and in the future when it comes to health care. Some problems are real, and some are perceived.

How Does Health Care Work in the United States?

Most people don't know that they pay for health care multiple times. If you think about it, everyone who works pays 1.45 % for Medicare. If your company has a health care plan, you may have to pay for part of the plan, which is the second way you pay for health care. If you pay income tax, you will find that part of your taxes go to pay for Medicaid. If you don't receive health care through your job, you may pay out of pocket, and then you still may have the aforementioned tax payments. The truth is the average person pays for health care three times.

Health Care in the United States is comprised of private and public health care providers who provide health care Services for a fee or for free. These services can be through hospitals, nursing homes, urgent care, doctors' offices, etc. The services that charge a fee for service are generally paid for using Medicare, Medicaid, private insurance/ACA, or cash. In general, a person will transfer his risk of illness or injury to an entity who agrees to pay for certain services. But how does this work, and how do Medicare, Medicaid, private insurance, and the ACA work?

There are five methods to pay for health care in the United States: the individual pays cash, the individual has private insurance, the individual has Medicaid, the individual has Medicare, and the ACA. Each of these methods is paid for differently, and each has different rules that govern how they pay, how much they pay, and how they manage risk. The health care system in the United States is based on these methods of payment and how they are funded.

Medicare

Medicare is health insurance for the following:

- people sixty-five or older
- people under sixty-five with certain disabilities
- people of any age with end-stage renal disease (ESRD) (permanent kidney failure requiring dialysis or a kidney transplant)

What Are the Different Parts of Medicare?

(Medicare.gov)

Medicare Part A (Hospital Insurance)

Medicare Part A helps cover the following:

- inpatient care in hospitals
- skilled nursing facility care
- hospice care
- home health care

You usually don't pay a monthly premium for Part A coverage if you or your spouse paid Medicare taxes while working. This is sometimes called premium-free Part A. If you aren't eligible for premium-free Part A, you may be able to buy Part A and pay a premium.

Medicare Part B (Medical Insurance)

Medicare Part B helps cover the following:

- services from doctors and other health care providers
- outpatient care
- home health care
- durable medical equipment
- some preventive services

Most people pay the standard monthly Part B premium. You can choose to buy a Medicare supplement insurance (Medigap) policy from a private company.

Note: You may want to get coverage that fills gaps in original Medicare coverage.

Medicare Part C (Medicare Advantage):

- run by Medicare-approved private insurance companies
- includes all benefits and services covered under Part A and Part B
- usually includes Medicare prescription drug coverage (Part D) as part of the plan
- usually includes extra benefits and services, in some cases for an extra cost

Medicare Part D (Medicare prescription drug coverage):

- run by Medicare-approved private insurance companies
- helps cover the cost of prescription drugs
- may help lower your prescription drug costs and help protect against higher costs in the future

Medicare Analysis

Medicare covers a lot but is not for everybody. Medicare is basically an 80-20 plan. Medicare shares risk with the individual and insurance companies. In general, the federal government pays 80% of the charge for a service provided, and the other 20% is covered by the person, Medicaid, or insurance. It is run by the federal government, and it is funded mostly by contributions that people make while they are working prior to hitting age sixty-five. The beauty of this program is they cap the risks and pass it to the individual or the insurance companies. There is no unlimited risk to the federal government to pay for illnesses or accidents. Medicare's origins stem from the inability of insurance companies to cover the elderly.

Medicare costs about $10,000 per person covered per year (about 60 million are enrolled with a budget of about $610 billion in 2017) or almost double the cost of private insurance before the ACA. There are a few reasons that Medicare is so expensive. First, Medicare covers people who are or will be in the last year of their lives where up to 31% of all health care expenses are incurred (https://www.ncbi.nlm.nih.gov/pmc/articles/PMC1464043/). Second, Medicare has tremendous administrative costs, between 6–8% of their budget (https://www.manhattan-institute.org/html/comparing-public-and-private-health-insurance-would-single-payer-system-save-enough-cover).

The fact is, if we were to utilize Medicare to be the basis of a health care system to cover all 330 million or so people in the United States, it would cost more than $3.3 trillion (based on 2017 enrollment of about 60 million with the budget for Medicare of $609 billion). The estimate to cover everyone on Medicare is interesting because some people with chronic illnesses are on Medicare, but because the population on Medicare may not reflect the entire population, the cost to cover everyone could be higher.

One of the biggest problems that people see in Medicare is what happens to people who run out of coverage from it and make too much money to qualify for Medicaid. These people often run through all their assets to pay for care before Medicaid will pick up the remainder of the care for the rest of their lives. So that person will have one standard of care while on Medicare and will essentially go bankrupt before getting on Medicaid, having a lower standard of care.

Medicare is similar to most health care systems around the world. In general, most health care systems around the world that are run by the government don't cover all illnesses or 100% of the cost of a procedure or service. In some cases, the services of the government plan are supplemented by private insurance. Insurance is mandated in most countries around the world.

MEDICAID

Medicaid is a joint federal and state program that helps with medical costs for some people with limited income and resources. Medicaid may also cover services not normally covered by Medicare, like long-term supports and services and personal-care services. Each state has different rules about eligibility and applying for Medicaid. If you qualify for Medicaid in your state, you automatically qualify for extra help, paying your Medicare prescription drug coverage (Part D). (www.medicaid.gov)

Your eligibility for Medicaid may depend on the following:

- your age
- whether you're pregnant
- whether you're blind
- if you have other disabilities
- whether you're a U.S. citizen

Certain legal immigrants may also be eligible.

If Medicaid covers a woman's labor and delivery, her baby may be covered for up to one year without needing to apply. People with Medicaid who are disabled or elderly also may get coverage for services like nursing home care or home- and community-based services.

The Medicaid program is jointly funded by the federal and state governments. The federal government pays states for a specified percentage of program expenditures, called the Federal Medical Assistance Percentage (FMAP).

FMAP varies by state based on criteria such as per capita income. The regular average state FMAP is 57%, but ranges from 50% in wealthier states up to 75% in states with lower per capita incomes (the maximum regular FMAP is 82%).

FMAPs are adjusted for each state on a three-year cycle to account for fluctuations in the economy. The FMAP is published annually in the Federal Register.

States must ensure they can fund their share of Medicaid expenditures for the care and services available under their state plan. Recognized sources of funding for the state share of Medicaid payments include the following:

- legislative appropriations to the single state agency
- intergovernmental transfers (IGTs)
- certified public expenditures (CPEs)
- permissible taxes and provider donations

Before CMS approves a state plan amendment, they must verify that state funding sources meet statutory and regulatory requirements so they can authorize federal financial participation (FFP) for the covered services.

Service Delivery and Provider Payment Rates

States can establish their own Medicaid provider payment rates within federal requirements. States generally pay for services through fee-for-service or managed-care arrangements.

Under fee-for-service arrangements, states pay providers directly for services. States may develop their payment rates based on the following:

- the costs of providing the service
- a review of what commercial payers pay in the private market
- a percentage of what Medicare pays for equivalent services

Under managed care arrangements, states contract with organizations to deliver care through networks and pay providers. Approximately 70% of Medicaid enrollees are served through managed-care delivery systems, where providers are paid on a monthly capitation payment rate.

Payment rates are often updated based on specific trending factors, such as the Medicare Economic Index or a Medicaid-specific trend factor

---

that uses a state-determined inflation adjustment rate. The methodologies for service rates are described in the Medicaid state plan.

How States Change Their Payment Methodology

To change the way they pay Medicaid providers, a state must submit a State Plan Amendment (SPA) for CMS to review and approval. Before the amendment's effective date, the state must also issue a public notice of the change. The notification is intended to widely inform providers and other stakeholders of changes to Medicaid payment rates.

CMS Review of Reimbursement Methodologies

CMS reviews state plan amendment reimbursement methodologies for consistency with the Social Security Act and other federal statutes and regulations.

This section requires that states "assure that payments are consistent with efficiency, economy and quality of care and are sufficient to enlist enough providers so that care and services are available under the plan at least to the extent that such care and services are available to the general population in the geographic area."

Medicaid Analysis

Medicaid has been expanded by the ACA, so it will cover people with incomes below 138% of the poverty line, currently just below $17,000. There are about 76 million people on Medicaid at a cost of about $580 billion. This is pure and easy for the individual. The individual has no risk and no obligation for the most part. The states cover about $210 billion in charges, and the federal government covers about $370 billion. Medicaid pays for people to go and get care.

For the most part, people go to a provider and the government pays. If you look at Medicaid from the point of view of the insured, it is as simple as if you get sick, go to the hospital or doctor and Medicaid pays. (That is a bit oversimplified, but you get the idea). On the flip side, Medicaid pays where Medicare leaves off and has unlimited risk to pay for the expenses of those covered. Medicaid can decline a service or procedure and has a payment schedule for reimbursements.

If we used the current version of Medicaid to service everyone, it would cost about $2.5 trillion per year. However, there could be no deductibles and no copays for the insured.

Medicaid is pure for the people who are serviced. The quality of care is basic but covers everything. It picks up when Medicare ends and takes care of the poor. Because it is jointly paid for by state and federal governments, there is significant administrative cost, waste, and fraud.

Private Insurance

Definition of *health insurance*:

A type of insurance coverage that pays for medical and surgical expenses that are incurred by the insured. Health insurance can either reimburse the insured for expenses incurred from illness or injury or pay the care provider directly. Health insurance is often included in employer benefit packages as a means of enticing quality employees (http://www.investopedia.com/terms/h/healthinsurance.asp).

Private Insurance Analysis

Private insurance was the payment mechanism for 46% of the people covered in the United States before the ACA. After the ACA, the health insurance companies joined forces with the government to cover those people without coverage. Some people choose to pay for private insurance out of pocket, and some people have private insurance as a benefit of their employment. As mentioned before, private insurance companies are interested in limiting risk to themselves while providing payment for health services for their clients.

There are many types of coverage, which range from catastrophic, high-deductible insurance that covers only serious illnesses or injury, to what are commonly called Cadillac plans that cover just about everything with low or no deductible.

Private insurance is at the center of the whole health care debate in this country. The problem is that not everyone is covered and the insurance companies are not interested in providing coverage for a "reasonable" price to everyone. Therefore, things started to change back in the 1960s when it came to insurance coverage; the government stepped in and started providing coverage to the poor and the elderly. Now there is a call to cover everyone with some sort of insurance. If everyone in the country was put on private insurance, it would cost about $2.276 trillion per year ($6896 times 330 million people). This is a significant discount to the current cost of care.

Health insurance has a simple process. An insurance company signs up a bunch of people to pay into a pool of funds that will be used to pay for any procedures that are required by anyone in the pool. The quality of the pool is determined by the risk within the pool. Insurance companies have a concept of "adverse selection" that determines who will be included in the pool to lessen the risk of the pool. This means that people with preexisting conditions or a family history of certain illnesses are a risk to the pool and add extra cost. The smaller the percentage of people who are adversely selected, the lower the risk of the pool and the greater the possibility of profit.

The other side of this equation is that because most of the risk pools have excluded those who may be sick or could possibly be sick, increasing the number of people added to the pool will most likely include a higher possibility of sick people. Therefore, it may cost more to cover all of the people in the country. Essentially, people who are young and healthy will opt out of any program that costs more than self-insurance, and the sick will opt in. That will increase the cost of the pool, and the cost of care will increase across the board, thus confirming the law of diminishing marginal returns.

The Patient Protection and Affordable Care Act

About the Law

The Affordable Care Act puts consumers back in charge of their health care. Under the law, a new Patient's Bill of Rights gives the American people the stability and flexibility they need to make informed choices about their health.

Coverage

- Ends Preexisting Condition Exclusions for Children: Health plans can no longer limit or deny benefits to children under nineteen due to a preexisting condition.
- Keeps Young Adults Covered: If you are under twenty-six, you may be eligible to be covered under your parents' health plan.
- Ends Arbitrary Withdrawals of Insurance Coverage: Insurers can no longer cancel your coverage just because you made an honest mistake.
- Guarantees Your Right to Appeal: You now have the right to ask that your plan reconsider its denial of payment.

Costs

- Ends Lifetime Limits on Coverage: Lifetime limits on most benefits are banned for all new health insurance plans.
- Reviews Premium Increases: Insurance companies must now publicly justify any unreasonable rate hikes.
- Helps You Get the Most from Your Premium Dollars: Your premium dollars must be spent primarily on health care—not administrative costs.

Care

- Covers Preventive Care at No Cost to You: You may be eligible for recommended preventive health services. No copayment.
- Protects Your Choice of Doctors: Choose the primary care doctor you want from your plan's network.
- Removes Insurance Company Barriers to Emergency Services: You can seek emergency care at a hospital outside of your health plan's network.

Patient's Bill of Rights

(https://www.whitehouse.gov/files/documents/healthcare-fact-sheets/patients-bill-rights.pdf)

- Ban on Discriminating Against Kids with Pre-Existing Conditions

Before reform, tens of the thousands of families have been denied insurance each year for their children because of an illness or condition. With the Patient's Bill of Rights, plans cannot discriminate against kids with preexisting conditions. In 2014, no one seeking coverage can be discriminated against because of a preexisting condition.

- Ban on Insurance Companies Dropping Coverage

Before reform, insurance companies could cancel your coverage when you were sick and needed it most because of a simple mistake on your application. With the Patient's Bill of Rights, insurance companies are banned from cutting off your coverage due to an unintentional mistake on your application.

- Ban on Insurance Companies Limiting Coverage

Before reform, cancer patients and individuals suffering from other serious and chronic diseases were often forced to limit or go without treatment because of an insurer's lifetime limit on their coverage. With the Patient's Bill of Rights, insurance companies can no longer put a lifetime limit on the amount of coverage, so families can live with the security of knowing that their coverage will be there when they need it most. The use of annual limits has been restricted and banned completely since 2014.

- Ban on Insurance Companies Limiting Choice of Doctors

Before reform, insurance companies could decide which doctor you could go to. With the Patient's Bill of Rights, if you purchase or join a new plan, you have the right to choose your own doctor in your insurer network.

- Ban on Insurance Companies Restricting Emergency Room Care

Before reform, insurance companies could limit which emergency room you could go to or charge you more if you went out of network. With the Patient's Bill of Rights, if you purchase or join a new plan, those plans are banned from charging more for emergency services obtained out of network.

- Guarantee You a Right to Appeal

Before reform, when insurers denied you coverage or restricted your treatment, you were left with few options to repeal. With the Patient's Bill of Rights, if you purchase or join a new policy, you will be guaranteed the right to appeal insurance company decisions to an independent third party.

- Covering Young Adults on Parent's Plan

With the Patient's Bill of Rights, young adults will be allowed to remain on their parents' plan until their twenty-sixth birthday unless they are offered coverage at work. Up to 2.4 million young adults could gain affordable coverage through this provision of the new law.

- Covering Preventive Care with No Cost

With the Patient's Bill of Rights, if you join or purchase a new plan, you will receive recommended preventive care with no out-of-pocket cost. Services like mammograms, colonoscopies, immunizations, prenatal and new-baby care will be covered, and insurance companies will be prohibited from charging deductibles, copayments, or coinsurance.

The Patient Protection and Affordable Care Act Analysis

In a nutshell, the ACA is a deal between the government and the insurance companies to provide coverage for the people in the country who are not already covered by some form of health care. It forces the insurance companies to offer the uninsured coverage that meets the new standard that the government has made. The government will also offer subsidies to those who meet certain criteria to pay for this coverage. People who earn less than 138% of the poverty level will automatically be enrolled in Medicaid. This is a beautiful system that benefits those who have preexisting conditions. The rights of the people are put first, above the practices of the insurance companies.

This is the reason for this book. The ACA is supposed to cover about 20 million more citizens at a cost of about $250 billion per year. This is about $12,500 per person per year. It was proposed that the ACA would cover the 50 or so million people who are not covered by the government or private insurance, but the Congressional Budget Office estimates about 20 million will ultimately will be covered. It has eliminated lifetime caps in coverage, eliminated the ability of private insurance companies to deny coverage for preexisting conditions, and is supposed to lower the cost of insurance while raising the quality of insurance. If we used the ACA to cover everyone in the United States, the cost would be about $4.125 trillion (330 million people at $12,500).

There are a few issues with the ACA. First, it mandates that the risk pools accept sick people. This necessarily increases the cost of insurance. As mentioned before, the higher number of sick people in the pool, the higher the cost to cover the pool.

Second, the ACA taxes essential components of the system like medical devices. There is a special tax on medical devices above and beyond the normal corporate tax. This tax will be passed on to the consumer. This adds cost to the system.

Third, the ACA mandates that the insurance companies cover specific illnesses that may not have been covered before the ACA. This adds more cost because more illnesses are covered.

Fourth, the ACA eliminates the lifetime and yearly caps on coverage. Caps are a mechanism to lower risk and thus lower cost. The elimination of caps adds to the cost of the program.

Finally, under the ACA, the tax structure of the country was changed, and taxes were added to pay for the system. This leads to more times that a person pays for health care and makes the system more complicated for the average person. There are several more things that can be fixed in the ACA, but to list every problem and the solutions would take more pages than the pages than were printed in the law itself.

Before the ACA, insurance companies insured the average person for about $5,900 per year. After the ACA, the cost of private insurance has risen to more than $6,700 per person per year. This is a 14% increase in price over a three-year period. The increase in price is directly related to the Patient Bill of Rights and the change in risk mitigation.

The suggestion that we scrap the ACA and start with another plan is not wise. The ACA started down a path that has merit. The Patient Bill of Rights has great ideas. Some of these ideas are contained in the health care plans in other countries. This bill of rights protects the people from both the insurance companies and, in theory, the government.

Medicare for All

In the past few years, there is a movement toward Medicare for all. The plan is being pushed by Bernie Sanders and many Democratic socialists. The plan would create a single-payer health care system in the United States that promises to provide comprehensive health care for everyone. According to Bernie Sanders,

> We outspend all other countries on the planet and our medical spending continues to grow faster than the rate of inflation. Creating a single, public insurance system will go a long way towards getting health care spending under control. The United States has thousands of different health insurance plans, all of which set different reimbursement rates across different networks for providers and procedures resulting in high administrative costs. Two patients with the same condition may get very different care depending on where they live, the health insurance they have and what their insurance covers. A patient may pay different amounts for the same prescription depending solely on where the prescription is filled. Health care providers and patients must navigate this complex and bewildering system wasting precious time and resources.
>
> By moving to an integrated system, the government will finally have the ability to stand up to drug companies and negotiate fair prices for the American people collectively. It will also ensure the federal government can track access to various providers and make smart investments to avoid provider shortages and ensure communities can access the providers they need. (https://live-berniesanders-com.pantheonsite.io/issues/medicare-for-all/)

There are a few inherent problems with the single-payer system that is proposed by Bernie Sanders. First, he is planning to eliminate the entire health Insurance industry. On the surface, the elimination of insurance companies may seem like a good idea; however, eliminating 2.66 million jobs and an industry that has more than $3 trillion in annual revenues would be catastrophic. Some may say that the insurance companies are evil and overcharge. However, this is a system that has managed health care in the United States for the past hundred or so years. It also has managed one of the most effective systems in the world.

Second, the system that Bernie Sanders is proposing will negotiate prices and schedule payments for doctors. Currently, under Medicare and Medicaid reimbursements, doctors can receive as little as $30 per doctor visit. If this is the payment that doctors can expect for services, the income for doctors will decrease. This most likely will lower the cost of doctors; however, in the long term, it will discourage students from becoming doctors. If doctors had a choice, they would stop accepting people on the single-payer system and only accept insurance plans that paid the price the doctor would charge. Currently, general practitioners in the United States earn an average of $161,000 compared to about $116,000 for general practitioners in the UK.

Third, the system fixes prices that creates shortages. In this situation, a shortage is nothing more than an excess demand for health care or pharmaceuticals that exceeds the available supply. This is the same problem that is plaguing the health care systems in the UK and Canada. There are more people that demand service than doctors to see them. This leads to longer wait times to get appointments and procedures.

"As a patient, all you need to do is go to the doctor and show your insurance card. Bernie's plan means no more copays, no more deductibles, and no more fighting with insurance companies when they fail to pay for charges" (https://live-berniesanders-com.pantheonsite.io/issues/medicare-for-all/).

Fourth, because the system doesn't have any mechanism for managing risk or the potential of unlimited financial costs, there is no way to project the total cost of the program. When a person can get unlimited services, that adds demand to the system. When the demand increases and the supply stays the same, the prices necessarily rise.

———

WHY IS THE HEALTH CARE SYSTEM IN THE UNITED STATES FAILING?

The problem with the health care system in the United States is that it has too many solutions to address too many issues. The insurance companies are set up to pool resources within a risk pool to make a profit while serving the needs to the clients they accept. This means that they will not serve those who cannot pay, those who are sick, and those who are elderly. That is okay in the United States because the government decided that it will provide health care for the elderly by creating Medicare. For the most part, Medicare works similar to the universal health care systems around the world. In most countries, the government scheme pays 70 or 80% of health care costs incurred by the people, and the people have mandatory insurance to pick up the remaining percentage.

The next issue is that the poor couldn't afford health insurance, and neither could some of the elderly. That is when the government created Medicaid. That is the solution for the poor. But there are still people that don't quite fit into the categories that are covered. That is why the government once again steps in and provides the ACA. This plan is supposed to cover everyone else. The issue is that the cost of health care had risen to a point that it was not affordable and the government had to subsidize care.

The real problem with the health care system in the United States is that everyone has an opinion and a solution that they say will fix the system. However, most of the solutions are more of the same, just with a few tweaks. Most of the solutions never take into account the effect of inflation, innovation, fraud, waste, payment risk, and economics. But the biggest problem is that most of the proposals don't take into account the effect of *cost*! Cost cannot be controlled by price fixing.

There are other incredibly complex issues that face the health care industry. Some people are getting healthier, and others have one or more chronic illnesses. The instances of type 2 diabetes is growing not just in the United States but also around the world. The pharmaceutical companies have been developing new drugs, but the cost of insulin has been skyrocketing. The cost of developing new drugs has not decreased, and lawsuits against pharmaceutical companies continue to make drugs more expensive.

The big question that needs to be answered is, "Why does the country continue to add another health care solution to the solutions that are already failing?" If insurance companies can't cover everyone, they may need to go. If Medicare and Medicaid can't fix the 8% administration cost and the 30% fraud and waste, maybe they need to go. If the ACA continues to cost 25% more than Medicare and increases the average cost of health insurance, maybe it needs to go. The fact is that each of the health care payment mechanisms in the United States have great attributes and, perhaps with some fixing, could serve the entire nation for about the same price that is paid around the world.

How Does Health Care Work in Other Countries?

Health care in other countries is not at all how we perceive it in the United States. The way some of the single-payer systems in Europe and around the world are presented to the public in the United States lead people to believe that the government pays everything and the people are taken care of 100%. Health care in these countries costs about half of the cost in the United States, but how are they really being paid for, and are the people in those countries paying more or less than the people in the United States?

Health Care Expenditures as Percent of GDP		Per-capita Spending ($USD)	Public Expenditure on Health, Percent of Total
Belgium	11.0%	$3,995	27.9%
Brazil	8.4%	$606	79.9%
Canada	10.4%	$4,079	70.2%
China	4.7%	$108	67.9%
France	11.4%	$3,696	77.8%
Germany	10.9%	$3,737	76.8%
Luxembourg	6.8%	$4,237	84.1%
Mexico	6.4%	$852	46.9%
Portugal	10%	$2,108	70.6%
Switzerland	11.2%	$4,627	59.1%

UK	10.1%	$3,129	82.6%
United States	17.6%	$8,086	46.5%

The above chart shows health care expenditures around the world in 2011, before the ACA. It is from the survey of health care that Deloitte did in 2011. Things have changed in the United States and the UK since then, but the chart is important because it shows the differences between how much is spent in each country in the study.

The important part of the chart is the right side where it shows "Public Expenditure on Health, Percent of Total." You can see that in the United States, the government picks up about 46% of health care expenses. That is about the same as the insurance companies. The insurance companies pick up about 46% of health care costs. The remaining 8% is paid in various ways, from people paying out of pocket to charities and free clinics picking up the tab. The interesting thing is that there is no government that is picking up 100% of the cost of health care. This is not even true in the UK where supposedly the government pays for everything. The fact is that no government pays 100% of health care costs. Each country has a different scheme that they use to serve their citizens.

It is crucial to know how each country runs their health care schemes to know what they do the best that may be implemented in the United States to improve our system. Because France and the UK were profiled in the movie *Sicko*, it seemed like explaining their schemes would be helpful in learning how to fix the system in the United States. The best systems in the world will be examined and the best features will be highlighted.

FRANCE

According to Michael Moore and his movie *Sicko*, everyone in France is giddy over their health care. In France, the government covers 100% of the people with health care. But how does their system work, and why were they number one in the world in health care according to the WHO in 2000?

SHI is financed by employer and employee payroll taxes (50%), a national earmarked income tax (35%), taxes levied on tobacco and alcohol, the pharmaceutical industry, and voluntary health insurance companies (13%), and state subsidies (2%).

"The healthcare system in France is funded partially by obligatory social security contributions (*sécurité sociale*), which are usually deducted from your salary. In 2016 employees paid around 8 percent in total, while employers paid around 13 percent of salary towards health costs. When you see a doctor or have medical treatment a percentage of the cost—usually about 70 percent of doctors' fees and 80 percent of hospital costs—will be reimbursed for most people through the French healthcare system, so long as you are referred by your 'attending doctor'. In the case of some major or long-term illnesses, 100 per cent of the costs are covered.

The remainder of your charge must be paid for either by the patient or through any supplementary private health insurance. This is why many people take out top-up health insurance (*l'assurance complémentaire santé*) often organised by a "mutual society" (*mutelle)*, or insurance provider. When you take out one of these policies, note that some may not cover certain sports and they may not offer immediate cover either. There are also other small charges that must be paid for by the patient, for example, a EUR 1 out-of-pocket charge per GP visit. (http://www.expatica.com/fr/healthcare/french-healthcare-france-health-care-system_101166.html#FRhealthcare)

In France, it is mandatory that everyone have health insurance. Not all chronic illnesses are covered, and insurance is needed to guarantee payment of costs that are not covered by the government. Those making less than about 10,000 euros do not pay the 8% tax. It is reserved for those who make over 10,000 euros.

In essence the French manage risk by, first, making sure that everyone is on the system, second, having a backup payment plan (insurance companies) to cover what is left of costs after government payments, and third, limiting what is covered by the government. What is interesting about the French system is the fact that companies pay 13% of their employees' wages to support the system. In the United States, companies match 1.45% of the employees' wages for Medicare, and there is an employer mandate under the ACA that can cost as much as 5.5% of an employee's salary. However, this is not close to 13%. For everyone in France who makes over about $14,000, 21% of their wages goes to support health care. As you can see, the cost of health care in France is borne mostly by the corporations and the people. As mentioned, the government picks up about 70% of costs, but not everything is covered (http://international.commonwealthfund.org/countries/france/).

The system in France can be thought of as a large-scale Medicare for all. The important difference between the system in the United States and the system in France is that risk in the United States is based on the individual and the cost to the individual is based on his/her risk. In France, the risk is not based on the risk of the individual. It is based on the individual's ability to pay. Those who make more pay more, and those who make less than about 10,000 euros pay nothing. This will become a theme as other countries are analyzed.

THE UK

Up until about 2012, the UK had a point-of-service single-payer health care system. The cost of the health care system became expensive to the government, so over a five-year period, the system was changed to allow for more privatization. "The NHS provides or pays for preventive services, including screening, immunization, and vaccination programs; inpatient and outpatient hospital care; physician services; inpatient and outpatient drugs; clinically necessary dental care; some eye care; mental health care, including some care for those with learning disabilities; palliative care; some long-term care; rehabilitation, including physiotherapy (e.g., after-stroke care); and home visits by community-based nurses" (http://international.commonwealthfund.org/countries/england/).

"Outpatient prescription drugs are subject to a copayment (currently GBP8.40, or USD12.14, per prescription item in England); drugs prescribed in NHS hospitals are free. NHS dentistry services are subject to copayments of up to GBP233.70 (USD338.00) per course of treatment. These charges are set nationally by the Department of Health" (http://international.commonwealthfund.org/countries/england/).

The health care system in the UK is promoted as a "free" system. It is actually paid for by taxes. The tax begins at about 182 pounds per week and is based on the class of insurance that you fall under. In general, a person will pay 12% of his salary in taxes to support the health care system. There is an additional tax of 2% if the income exceeds 892 pounds per week. Companies also have a tax to pay to support the health care system. In general, the tax that a company will pay based on an employee salary is 13.8% (https://www.gov.uk/national-insurance-rates-letters).

In the UK currently, the old point-of-service system has been changed. For most of the people, things are the same; however, the new system has more private doctors and hospitals. Eleven percent of the population now has private insurance that allows them to get faster service at private hospitals and doctors. Those with special needs for costly or large amounts of prescription drugs pay a monthly charge. "An estimated 548 private hospitals and between 500 and 600 private clinics in the U.K. offer a range of services, including treatments either unavailable in the NHS or subject to long waiting times, such as bariatric surgery and fertility treatment, but generally do not have emergency, trauma, or intensive-care facilities. Private providers must be registered with the Care Quality Commission and with NHS Improvement, but their charges to private patients are not regulated, and there are no public subsidies" (http://international. commonwealthfund.org/countries/england/).

This is not the same health care scheme that the UK had in 2012 where everything was government run and the health care providers were government employees.

Japan

Japan is very similar to France in the way that they run their health care scheme. The citizens in Japan can use any health care facility in Japan and pay 30% of the charge. The government picks up the 70%. It is mandatory that everyone have private insurance. This insurance is the reimbursement for the 30% for which the people are responsible. The state health insurance is 9.90% and is split equally between the employer and the employee. For those who are seventy-five years and older or are over the age of sixty-five with a registered disability, the Long Life Medical Care System (*chôju iryô seido*) is applicable. Those older than seventy-five have a 10% copayment rather than the 30% that is paid by those who are younger.

National Health Insurance (NHI), on the other hand, is for those who are under the age of seventy-five and unemployed, self-employed (including contractors), or retired, as well as the dependent family members of those just mentioned.

Just like the EHI, the NHI covers 70% of your hospital bills. To apply, you must visit the Residential Affairs Division at your local city or ward office. The premium is based on your age and your previous year's income. There is a cap to the amount of health Insurance tax that is paid at 1,355,000 JPY as of April 2018. For average salaries of 1,355,000 JPY and above, the standard salary is 1,390,000 JPY.

Managed by your local government, the premium fees and insurance coverage depends on the insured's income. For low-income individuals, the insurance may cover up to 90% of all medical bills while for others, the standard 70% applies.

GERMANY

Germany had the first state-sponsored health care system in the world. It started in 1883 and covered about 10% of the citizens. Now the German health care system serves about 86% of its citizens through its statutory health insurance. Insurance is mandatory in Germany; however, there is an option that allows those making more than $67,000 to pay for private insurance. About 11% of the population has taken this option.

The statutory health insurance covers inpatient, outpatient, mental health, and prescription drug coverage. It is administered through what are called sickness funds. The sickness funds are run by over a hundred nongovernmental organizations that compete for business. The sickness funds are funded by the government. The government collects a payroll tax of 14.6%, which is split evenly between the employer and employee.

Within Germany's legal framework, the federal government has wide-ranging regulatory power over health care but is not directly involved in care delivery. The Federal Joint Committee, which is supervised by the Federal Ministry of Health, determines the services to be covered by sickness funds. To the extent possible, coverage decisions are based on evidence from comparative-effectiveness reviews and health technology (benefit-risk) assessments.

The Federal Association of Sickness Funds works with the Federal Association of Statutory Health Insurance Physicians and the German Hospital Federation to develop the ambulatory care fee schedule for sickness funds and the diagnosis-related group (DRG) catalog, which are then adopted by bilateral joint committees. Germany's state governments also play an important administrative role. The 16 state governments determine hospital capacity and finance hospital investments. States also supervise public health services. (https://www. commonwealthfund.org/international-health-policy-center/ countries/germany)

The German system is overseen by the government in conjunction with nongovernment entities. The government doesn't get involved with the actual service, but polices the system and provides funding through taxes. The nongovernment entities determine the fees that will be charged throughout the system.

The German system is very different from the rest of the world. Even though insurance is mandatory, the country has an opt-out option for those who make enough money to afford private insurance. In most countries around the world, there is a division between the government-provided health care and private insurance that picks up where the government leaves off. In Germany, the sickness funds cover almost all of the cost of illnesses (there are copayments and deductibles that are set by the sickness funds).

CANADA

In Canada, there is a perception that health care is free. That is not really the case. In most countries around the world, citizens pay for health care through a payroll tax or some sort of value-added tax. In Canada, the health care system is run by the thirteen provinces, and the funds come from taxes both at the country and provincial levels. Because of the way the system is administered by thirteen different provinces, there are differences from province to province. That being said, there are some services that are not covered throughout the entire system. Canada does not cover dental services, physiotherapy, psychologist visits, chiropractic care, and cosmetic, or plastic surgery. Furthermore, illegal aliens are not covered under the Canadian system.

> To qualify for federal financial contributions, Provincial and Territorial (p/t) insurance plans must provide first-dollar coverage of medically necessary physician, diagnostic, and hospital services (including inpatient prescription drugs) for all eligible residents. All P/T governments also provide public health and prevention services (including immunizations) as part of their public programs.

> However, there is no nationally defined statutory benefit package; most public coverage decisions are made by P/T governments in conjunction with the medical profession. Because of this, coverage varies across P/T insurance plans for services not federally mandated as medically necessary, including outpatient prescription drugs, mental health care,

vision care, dental care, home care, midwifery services, medical equipment, and hospice care.

Most provinces have public prescription drug coverage programs for specific populations, such as recipients of social assistance, seniors aged 65 and older, and children and youth. Some programs charge premiums, often income-related. (https://www.commonwealthfund.org/international-health-policy-center/countries/canada)

There was a study done in 2015 by the Fraser Institute (https://www.fraserinstitute.org/?id=23178) that addresses how much is paid in taxes by Canadian citizens. They broke down the funding for the Canadian health care scheme into ten tax brackets. The average amount paid per person was about $4,000. However, those with the lowest incomes paid about $500 per year, and those with the highest incomes paid upward of $59,000.

The Canadian health care scheme works as a point-of-service system. Citizens go to a hospital or clinic and receive service without a payment. There is no deductible or copayment.

Summary

This is just a cross section of countries around the world and how they administer health care schemes. The vast majority of countries run systems that cover most illnesses and preventative care. The goal of every country is to serve as close to 100% cf the citizens with health care. This is generally achieved by mandating that everyone pay into a government-administered system and hold a supplemental private health insurance plan for what is not covered. In general, the funding mechanism is a payroll tax that is split between the employer and employee. The payment mechanism is generally reimbursement through insurance companies and the government entity responsible for health care.

There are aspects of each system that allow it to function effectively and efficiently. This project has taken those aspects and utilized them to develop a plan for the United States that will meet the goals of the World Health Organization and make the United States the number one health care system in the world.

PART II

The Philosophy of Designing a Health Care System

THE CURIOSITY ISSUE

In 2009, NASA was in the process of designing the Mars rover *Curiosity*. *Curiosity* was supposed to be sent to Mars in 2011. The mission seemed easy enough: design a vehicle that could be sent to Mars and land it on the Red Planet. Then after landing, the rover would survey Mars and send back information to NASA. Before the mission could be launched, each component and process had to be tested. The cost of the project was more than $5 billion, so every process was critical.

While NASA was testing the parachute that would be deployed to slow the decent of the rover through the Martian atmosphere, there was an issue. When the parachute was deployed, it turned inside out and ripped to shreds. To fix the problem, NASA reevaluated the issue and determined that the rover would be traveling about 900 miles per hour through the atmosphere on a planet with an atmospheric density about one-tenth of the Earth's. Furthermore, the gravity on Mars is about one-thirteenth of the gravity on Earth. This presented a problem. How do you test a parachute on Earth that is supposed to function on Mars when conditions are not the same?

NASA did some calculations and determined that they could deploy the parachute in a wind tunnel with winds about 90 miles per hour. The initial experiments were successful. However, on a few experiments, the parachute failed. This meant that there was a possibility that there would be a failure on Mars. This could not happen. This failure was repeated on several other trials.

Because of this issue and a few other issues, the Mars mission was delayed for about two years. It was found that on Earth, the velocity of the wind allowed time for the parachute to deploy and tangle. It was not the same as the deployment on Mars. On Mars, the parachute would not have time to tangle and turn inside out, destroying itself. This observation allowed NASA to continue to push the *Curiosity* mission forward.

Why Is Health Care So Expensive in the United States?

The development of the *Curiosity* was chosen to illustrate the complexities of developing and implementing a plan from scratch. The cost of *Curiosity* at $5 billion was huge compared to the $17 billion total budget of NASA in 2009. It is larger than the percentage of health care to the U.S. GDP. That is why it was so crucial to get it right. A $5 billion failure would destroy the credibility of NASA. Health care is 17% of the U.S. GDP, and to design a system that fails would be catastrophic, especially because the government would continue to run that scheme for years even with the failure.

What does the *Curiosity* experiment tell us about the health care systems around the world compared to the health care system in the United States? The United States has more than double the population of Russia and almost four times the population of Germany. The United States has a population at least four times than that of almost every country in the world that has a health care system. In some cases, the population in the United States is more than fifteen times the population of some countries with government-run health care. The economy of the United States is more than triple than that of most countries that have government-run or universal health care. When you compare the United States to the world, the comparison starts to look like the comparison of Earth to Mars in the *Curiosity* case. In some cases, health care in the countries with universal health care have costs that when compared to the United States make it a poor comparison. The average general practitioner in the UK makes about $116,000 compared to $161,000 for the United States. This is one of the costs that necessarily raises the expense of the U.S. health care system. There is the same type of correlation for the average income in the United States and the rest of the world.

It is easy to know why health care costs more in the United States than in every other country in the world. It is the cost of living. The median salary in the United States is about $56,000, and the average salary in the United States is about $80,000. In the UK, the average salary is about $40,000. There is no country in Europe where average salaries are higher or the same as in the United States. On the other hand, most of the countries in Europe have average salaries that are less than our proposed $15 per hour minimum wage.

Looking at the basic costs of health care, you find the price of a doctor's visit is one of the factors in the cost of health insurance. The price of a doctor's visit is driven by the doctor's expectation of what his salary should be for the year. If you compare the salaries of doctors in other countries to the salaries in the United States, the comparison makes the difference in cost for health care quite clear. As mentioned earlier, the salary for a general practitioner in the UK is $45,000 less than a GP in the United States. This is about a 39% difference. Perhaps this means that the cost of health care in the United States necessarily has to be at least 39% higher than in the UK.

Issues

One of the biggest issues that the United States has when it comes to health care is the desire to fix the system. One example of this is Medicare and Medicaid. Medicare was implemented because the insurance companies had an aversion to covering people over sixty-five years old. Medicaid was implemented because the poor couldn't afford health insurance. According to the GAO, the administrative costs of these programs is about 8% of their budgets. Furthermore, according to a speech given by Barack Obama, there is about 30% fraud and waste in Medicare and Medicaid. This means that based on 2018 budgets, about $400 billion is spent before any person receives medical care from Medicare and Medicaid.

These government programs operate on a reimbursement basis. They reimburse the health care provider for the services provided. This reimbursement is lower than the provider would normally accept. Because of this, the providers have to adjust the cost of service for those paying with insurance or out-of-pocket higher to achieve the desired average compensation. In the case of the ACA, the government had a desire to generate revenue from the health care system, so they issued taxes on components of the system. There was a tax on insurance companies and medical device companies that necessarily raised the cost of health care. Furthermore, the ACA eliminated the ability of insurance companies to lower costs through a system of raising premiums or denying service to those who are adversely selected. The program made it illegal to reject a patient because of a preexisting condition. The issue is that there was not a corresponding influx of healthy patients to offset this added cost.

Payment risk is another huge cost to the health care system. Before the ACA, there was about 16% of the population that was not covered by some sort of health care payment scheme. These people had to pay cash for all health care services. The effect of this issue was that when people got sick or injured, they would show up at a hospital, and the hospital was mandated to serve them. In some cases, the person didn't have the resources to pay the hospital, and the hospital had to sell the bad debt or just accept the default. The nonpayment to hospitals, dentists, eye doctors, and general practitioners is the reason that some hospitals have $90 boxes of tissues. This is the reason that there is cost in health care that is not assigned to the government or insurance companies. This cost is handled by the health care providers and manifests itself in higher prices for products and services. This cost can be as high as 5% of the cost for hospitals (https://www.usatoday.com/story/news/politics/2017/07/03/who-pays-when-someone-without-insurance-shows-up-er/445756001/).

Managing Costs and payments are where flaws rest in most government programs around the world. The cost of health care in the United States was about $2.7 trillion before the ACA and is about $3.3 trillion today. How is that handled? The average working person with company-sponsored health insurance, assuming the policy held was pre-ACA, the person would most likely split the cost of his/her policy 50-50 with the company which he/she works. The policy may cost $600 per month. That means that the person pays $300 per month, and the company pays $300 per month. Sadly, that is not the end. The person is mandated to pay 1.45 % of his/her salary for Medicare that he/she may get at some point in the future. Not the end yet, the company matches the contribution to Medicare. That is not the end yet. The person then pays a small part of his taxes to support Medicaid and the ACA.

If you look at this critically, you find that each person who has company-sponsored health care pays once for the policy once for Medicare, once for Medicaid, and once for the ACA. Then the company pays for the policy once for Medicare and then taxes to pay for Medicaid and the ACA. Companies who provide health care pay three times for health care.

What happens if a person works and is on the ACA? The person pays for the policy and pays for Medicare and pays Medicaid and the ACA through taxes. Then the government subsidizes the insurance if the person qualifies. The person's employer, well, you know, they match the Medicare payment through taxes they pay for Medicaid and the ACA, and they may pay a penalty for not providing health insurance. Most people pay for health insurance at least three times. There is a price for insurance, a price for Medicare, a price for Medicaid, and a price for the ACA. All these prices are paid by the people, and most people only have the services of one. This is the first issue that must be addressed when the current system is replaced. The people should only pay once for health care.

Realities

The first thing that is important about health care is that there is a cost associated with providing care. While doing a search on health care in the UK, I found that the system is promoted as "free" health care for the citizens of the country. However, doing a search for how the services are paid, I found that there is a tax on the citizens who make more than £182 per week. This is the same concept with every health care system in the world, there is a cost to run the system that must be paid. Digging a little deeper, I discovered that caregivers must be paid, pharmaceutical companies must be paid, medical supplies companies must be paid, medical-device companies must be paid, hospitals must be paid. There is a long line of entities that must be paid.

The cost of the health care system in the United States in 2017 was about $3.3 trillion. What must happen when the current system is replaced is a method of payment that will provide enough revenue to fully fund the program. The system should not run deficits.

The cost of health care continues to rise not just in the United States but around the world as well. Since the institution of the ACA, the cost of health insurance has risen 46% in the United States. This rate is faster than the rate of inflation. This is one of the most important issues in health care. Before the ACA, the average individual paid about $5,900 per year for health insurance. In the years that the ACA has been operating, the cost of an individual health insurance policy has risen to about $6,700 per year.

The cost of the average insurance policy is the biggest problem that this country has. There is no way that a person who makes $20,000 per year can afford to pay this amount. There is no way that a person who makes $56,000, the median income, or the average income of $80,000 can afford to pay this.

Another reality is that the cost of taking care of a person with a chronic illness is more than the cost of taking care of a healthy person. Chronic illnesses like diabetes have been increasing around the world, and the cost of taking care of these people is increasing, causing an increase of cost to the health care systems around the world. The cost of insulin has increased by multiples in the past ten years.

Because of the rising amount of people with chronic illnesses like type 2 diabetes, the risk to the health insurance companies increases. The cost of health care in the United States is driven by risk. Health insurance companies have actuaries that figure out the risk of individuals and aggregate the risk to determine the cost of a policy to the individual in a risk pool. Insurance companies used to limit risk by limiting adverse selection, thus reducing the cost to the pool. With the Patient Bill of Rights, insurance companies now must accept those who would normally be adversely selected. This has raised costs to the insurance companies and caused the increase in premiums.

However, the biggest reality that stands in the way of designing a new health care system in the United States is not rooted in cost or risk or even various chronic illnesses. The biggest issues are social and political. It is easy to see that there are multiple plans to reform health care in the United States. Some Republicans want to provide health savings accounts. Some Democrats want a single-payer system like what they have in the UK or Canada. Some people follow Bernie Sanders and want Medicare for all. Some people believe that mandating that everyone be on one system will violate their rights to choose. Some people believe that the majority should be able to force everyone into a system that would benefit everyone and save money. Some people believe that health insurance companies are evil and should be done away with. Some people believe that the government is wasteful and should be excluded from running any health care system. These are huge issues. They are issues because some of these people who follow one philosophy or another are not willing to change their mind or accept another solution. That is the exact reason that 6.5 million people opted to pay a penalty rather than participate in the ACA. This means that to serve all the people, some people will have to have some sort of compensating differential or incentive to convince them to participate in the plan.

Economics

When asked about how he would handle health care, Economics Nobel Prize winner Milton Friedman stated, "I said before I do not believe you ought to have any special program for medicine at all. I believe I have long been in favor of substituting for our present whole set of welfare arrangements, a comprehensive negative income tax, which would provide to individuals below a level a sum of money, which would assure they would be able to maintain a particular level. There is no reason why part of that sum of money cannot be spent on the purchase of the same kind of medical insurance everybody else has . . . The problem of poverty is money. And we ought to have a program under which we assure a minimum level of income, of spending, and then let people spend it the way they want."

Milton Friedman is perhaps one of the greatest economists in the twentieth century. In his view, the cost of health care was not a real problem. The problem was that those who couldn't afford to pay for it just needed a small bit of help. There was no need to have a universal health care system, just a method to help the poor pay for health insurance or medicine as he said. This was the 1970s, just after the roll out of Kaiser Permanente. There is a glaring issue with his solution. Doctor Friedman would have also argued that the poor should be able to use the negative income tax on anything they wanted to purchase. If the poor didn't purchase health insurance, the issue is moot.

To start understanding some of the issues and offering solutions, economics is crucial. Economic concepts will show why the ACA was so expensive and failed. Furthermore, economics will explain the failings of some health care systems around the world and perhaps offer some solutions. One of the cost drivers of health care is prescription drugs. In Canada, one of the mechanisms that is used to lower the cost of health care is negotiating the cost of prescription drugs. Then the government subsidizes the cost of drugs to those who cannot afford them. This has the same effect as the Nixon wage and price freeze in 1970. Eventually the cost of oil was above the price that was being charged. This created a shortage. This type of price fixing is taking place all around the world in health care. The effect is the government bears the added cost of fixing prices. This manifests in deficits and increases the national debt.

The ACA promised to lower the cost of health care in the United States and save the average family $2,500 per year. However, there were several economic issues that stood in the way of this promise. One of the glaring issues was the tax on medical devices. When you tax a product, the result is that the manufacturer will shift the cost of the tax to the employee in lower wages and the consumer in higher prices. The ACA effectively caused the price of some of the products that are a cost to the system to become costlier. This added costs to the system and instead of lowering the cost of providing health care. It raised the cost. The ACA didn't account for added demand. It is a basic law of economics that if you increase the demand for a good or service while keeping the supply constant, the price will increase. There is no doubt that if the cost of health care increased because of added demand with the ACA, the cost of any new health care system that would service the needs of all the people in the United States will necessarily increase the cost of health care.

The ACA instituted a bill of rights that mandated that the insurance companies accept people with preexisting conditions. This was a benefit to sick people and/or people with chronic illnesses. The ACA also allowed young adults from eighteen to twenty-six to remain on their parents' insurance. However, it did not offset the greater risk of the chronically ill people with significantly more people who were healthy. Furthermore, it eliminated the benefit of charging people between the ages of eighteen to twenty-six. This changed the makeup of the risk pool and caused higher prices because adverse selection could no longer be used to mitigate risk.

Not all cost benefits for the people benefit the people. On the surface, it would seem that allowing young adults to remain on their parents' health insurance would be a benefit. However, this may not reduce cost to the system and thus may cost more to the consumer. One of the benefits to pooling risk is that those who are healthy offset the risk of those who have chronic illnesses. Generally, those between the ages of eighteen and twenty-six are healthy. If they remain in the risk pool on their parents' policy, there is no opportunity to have them pay into the pool and thus offset the cost of someone chronically ill. So those young adults become adversely selected because they are not paying into the pool but their risk to the pool is absolute. If those young adults were required to pay for health care, they would be a benefit to the pool as they are healthy, in general, and the risk of illness is less than someone with chronic illnesses. Therefore, the cost of the pool can be lower, and the cost savings can be passed on to everyone in the pool.

One of the biggest issues in health care today is the increase in the amount of people diagnosed with chronic illnesses like diabetes. In Japan, as mentioned earlier, the instances of diabetes have been increasing. This has led to increasing costs to take care of these people. The cost of insulin and other drugs have been increasing around the world. The question is, "Why is the price of insulin increasing around the world, and how can this be slowed or reversed?"

The simple answer is supply and demand. Understanding supply and demand is the key to lowering cost in any economic system. Type 2 diabetes has been increasing around the world. Because of that, the demand for insulin and other diabetes drugs has been increasing. The supply of insulin did not increase to handle the demand, so the prices rose. The pharmaceutical companies realized that they not just had to build capacity but there was also an opportunity to develop other drugs that would be instrumental in treating diabetes. That meant that there would be more research and development. That added cost into the system. To lower the demand for diabetes drugs, the number of people with type 2 diabetes must be reduced. The solution could be as simple as a change in diet and exercise. That may seem like a simple answer; however, in the United States, the diet of thirty million people who, in general, qualify for Medicaid is based on the SNAP program that may have to be changed to accommodate better diets. This could add costs to a different part of the United States economy.

Another of the large economic issues is inflation. The cost of health care is growing faster than inflation in the United States. This must be addressed. In 2011, the total cost of health care was $2.7 trillion. By 2017, the cost had grown to $3.3 trillion. What happened is that the ACA forced the insurance companies to cover those with preexisting conditions and took away the healthy people that would offset the risk. Furthermore, the ACA took a large amount of healthy people and dumped them into Medicaid, lowering the risk. Before the ACA, health insurance was less expensive on average than Medicare and Medicaid. After the ACA, private health insurance was more expensive than Medicaid. The total cost of health care increased by about 4% per year.

The way to look at the economics in planning a health care system is first to look at the issues and make sure that, when fixing any of the issues, there is no violation of any economic principles.

Building a Philosophy

The secret of change is to focus all of your energy, not on fighting the old, but on building the new.

—Socrates

There is no perfect health care system. The independent auditing company Deloitte did a worldwide survey in 2011 and found that there is dissatisfaction with every health care system around the world. The conclusion that can be drawn from this survey is building a new health care system is a difficult undertaking. The fact is in the United States, there are three things that stand in the way of achieving the goal of building a health care system that works for everyone and costs less: the Democrats, the Republicans, and the Constitution. There are several truths that have been discussed in previous sections. Before even starting an investigation on what works well in other countries or what works well in the United States, what can't be changed must be addressed.

There are several people who hate insurance companies and want to do away with them. On the other side of the equation, there are several people who want smaller government and will not approve of government-run health care. The health insurance companies have a huge lobby that is working toward keeping health insurance companies in business. There are a several people who will not vote to approve a plan that does not include abortion, and on the other side, there are a several people who will not sign up for a program that includes abortion and contraceptives. How can each of these groups be satisfied at the same time?

There is no way to make doctors take less money for their services. This should be obvious to everyone. The issue is nobody would want to be a doctor if there was no money in it, and people could sue for malpractice. There is no way to make companies sell medical supplies for less than it cost to produce them. This would put the medical supply companies out of business and cause shortages. There is no way to make medical device companies sell for less than it costs to produce their products. Same reason as above, there is no way to get pharmaceutical companies to sell at less than cost. In other words, there are costs that must be paid.

Comparing the costs of a product or service in the United States to other countries is also futile. The median income in the United States is about $56,000 compared to about $33,000 in the UK, $6,200 in China, $33,000 in Japan, and $30,000 in France. That means that the average salaries of doctors and nurses are going to be higher in the United States. The average salaries of the administration in doctors' offices and hospitals are going to be more expensive. This also means that it is necessary that the cost of health care products and services are going to be costlier in the United States than around the world.

The organization that ranks health care around the world, the Organisation for Economic Co-operation and Development (OECD), has an evaluation system that values low-cost systems over those that are expensive. This is one reason that the United States is ranked outside of the top 20 nations providing health care. The OECD also looks at the percentage of people who are covered by the health care scheme. This means that even if the cost of the health care system in the United States decreases by 25%, the country will still be judged lower because of the percentage of people who are outside of the system. The converse is also true: if everyone in the country is covered by some sort of health care scheme but the cost of the system is not significantly decreased, the country will most likely still be considered outside of the top 20 nations. The truth is that there is no way to lower the cost of health care significantly based on the costs of products and services without lowering the standard of living in the country. There is also no way to put everyone on one health care scheme without changing the mindset in the country.

Knowing how the rest of the world handles health care, I can offer a few things that can be taken from them and a few things that may not work in the United States. The first thing that must be understood is that something drastic would have to happen for the government of the United

States to take over all health care in the country and force all health care to be nonprofit. Judging from the performance of Medicare, Medicaid, and the ACA, I think most people would choose a different path. The second thing to note is that health care is about one-sixth of the economy, so to eliminate or destroy a large part of this system would be catastrophic. The third thing to note is that when the ACA was implemented, more people opted out than opted to be covered by the plan. If it weren't for the fact that 12 million people were put on Medicaid, the program would have only served about 11 million people with a goal of 20 million. That is a failure.

Currently in the United States, the bulk of the cost of health care is incurred by about 12% of the people, and the sickest 40% of the people account for 90% of all health care spending. These people have chronic illnesses. That means cancer, diabetes, hypertension, stroke, heart disease, pulmonary conditions, Alzheimer's disease, tooth decay, arthritis, and mental illnesses. To offset these people, there are about 50% of the people who use less than $250 of health care per year.

There is a way to classify the different types of users of health care in the United States. The easiest is to rank those who need health care the most to the least. You see, 40% of the people account for 90% of all health care spending. Those people need health care and will most likely opt for any health care that would allow them to shift their risk of illness to someone who would pay. However, there are 50% of the people who are not ill and have no expectation of illness. Some of these people would opt not to pay for health insurance or any health care plan because they feel they don't need it.

This is the difference between the United States and other countries. In other countries, for the most part, the government decides if health care is mandatory or if a person can opt out. In the United States, unless health care is a tax, the people have the right to decline to pay, and thus, health care cannot be made mandatory. This is the reason that 6.5 million people decided to pay a fine rather than pay for the ACA. This is also the reason that designing a system that serves 100% of the citizens of the United States is difficult and requires a compensating differential.

Ranking the likelihood of people who would pay for health care is important in putting together a new health care program that will serve everyone. The ACA could not fully cover the whole country. Some would say that was because the individual mandate was not included. The fact is that the Constitution would not allow a mandate. That is the issue: choice.

Identifying the people that are apt to select health care over nothing is key to knowing what type of compensating differential that must be offered. There must be a compensating differential that will convince everyone that they should pay for and carry some sort of health care coverage.

Breaking down the likelihood further, there are 12% of the population that will always choose to purchase health insurance or health care if it were affordable. These are the people who are chronically ill, especially those with more than one chronic illness. The second most likely group to purchase health care coverage are those who have one chronic illness or expect to have a chronic illness and are risk averse. These people make up close to all of the remaining 28% of the chronically ill who spend 90% of the health care dollars and some of those who are in good health but are just risk averse. There are some people who choose to pay for health insurance because their employer picks up some of the cost of the coverage.

There are also two types of people who will not purchase health care until they are sick or injured. Those are the people within the 50% who spend less than $250 per year and are not risk averse and those who refuse because of political philosophy. It becomes clear that only the last two groups need a compensating differential.

The problem with offering a compensating differential is that most of the time, the compensating differential is in the form of money. When it comes to the government, it is usually a tax incentive or a handout. The issue with a monetary compensating differential or "bribe" is that it becomes costly the more people that you have to "bribe." There must exist a method to administer health care that would allow health care to be the compensating differential. In other words, the benefit of having coverage would compensate for the price of the service, and everyone would opt to have coverage and pay for the service willingly.

Currently the number one ranked system in the world is Japan. Japan runs a scheme that is basically a 70-30 system that covers hospital and doctors' visits. Most people in Japan have private insurance because it is mandatory to pay the remaining 30% left after the government pays. France is a similar story. They have basically an 80-20 plan (they pay differently for dental and doctors' visits) with private insurance. It is interesting that there are about two countries that have a true single-payer system. Every other country that has national health care has a hybrid between national insurance and private insurance.

These systems are mandatory. That means that everyone must enroll and pay into the system (there are income exclusions). This means that none of these systems can be implemented in the United States because of choice. This is made clear by the experience with the individual mandate for the ACA. Six and a half million people opted out of carrying health care and paid a penalty, and more than twenty million didn't pay a fine and/or chose an alternative. When offered a plan that was supposed to cover the 16% of the population without insurance, more people opted not to use the new system. Now we are getting closer to discovering who we need to handle. This leads to the big question, "How can we develop a compensating differential that would convince everyone to pay for health care?"

The World Health Organization and the Framework

Because there has already been an exhausting discussion of the health care systems both in the United States and around the world and there has been an analysis of cost and risk, there is not going to be a huge exhausting philosophy in building the system. To start with, we are going to use the World Health Organization definition of *health* from 1946: "a state of complete physical, mental, and social well-being and not merely the absence of disease or infirmity" (http://www.who.int/governance/eb/who_constitution_en.pdf).

Then without reinventing the wheel, the foundation and goals of the health care system that will be built will be founded on the precepts of the World Health Organization.

The goal of universal health coverage is to ensure that all people obtain the health services they need without suffering financial hardship when paying for them.

For a community or country to achieve universal health coverage, several factors must be in place, including:

1. A strong, efficient, well-run health system that meets priority health needs through people-centered integrated care (including services for HIV, tuberculosis, malaria, non-communicable diseases, maternal and child health) by:

- informing and encouraging people to stay healthy and prevent illness;
- detecting health conditions early;
- having the capacity to treat disease; and
- Helping patients with rehabilitation.
2. Affordability – a system for financing health services so people do not suffer financial hardship when using them. This can be achieved in a variety of ways.
3. Access to essential medicines and technologies to diagnose and treat medical problems.
4. A sufficient capacity of well-trained, motivated health workers to provide the services to meet patients' needs based on the best available evidence.

It also requires recognition of the critical role played by all sectors in assuring human health, including transport, education and urban planning.

According to the World Health Organization, everyone deserves health care. (The issues with citizenship and other limitations will be discussed later.) But what can be done to coerce the people who would opt out of a system to opt in and pay for the service? If people opt out, how can health care be administered to the greatest number of people or all of the people?

BUILDING THE SYSTEM

We know what the WHO mandates and some of the issues that plague the current system. To start building a new system, the key is to break down the current system into its components. The United States health care system has two components: service and payment. If a person is ill or injured, they go to a medical service provider and receive treatment. According to the OECD, the service or treatment part of health care in the United States is not broken. The issue is the provider expects payment. We go back to the beginning and know that there are a bunch of methods of payment. This is the problem. In the United States, there are still between twenty and thirty million people who must pay with cash or have no method of payment.

In 2000, the United States was ranked thirty-seventh in the world in health care by the OECD, and the biggest reason for this ranking was the cost. The answer to the cost problem in the UK was to issue everyone a card and let them obtain what they need from the sources available. That would be incredible, but in the United States, it would also be incredibly expensive. The reason is that there would be no incentive for the health care providers to be honest with charges for services, and the payer would have unlimited liability for the charges. In other words, there would be a large amount of fraud and waste, more than the 30% we currently have in the government run systems.

In Japan, the government owns about 15% of the health care facilities, and the other 85% are nonprofit. They have taken away the profit motive. Japan has also put everyone on the same system so there is no competition and the people must play by the rules. In the UK, most of the providers are employees of the government. This means that there is no incentive to cheat the system. Basically, in most countries around the world, the health care providers are either nonprofit, employees of the government, or owned by the government. This is not the case in the United States.

According to former president Obama, there is about 30% fraud and waste in Medicare and Medicaid. This still has not been addressed. There is also fraud and waste in private insurance. To build an efficient and effective system, fraud and waste must be controlled.

In the United States, before the ACA, about 84% of the population was covered with some sort of health care system: Medicaid, Medicare, or private insurance. The health care providers in the United States are private, some for profit and some nonprofit. There are some who cheat the system and some who are honest. When the government or insurance companies catch those who cheat, they are punished, but not harshly enough to stop others from cheating. A new scheme would have to have a mechanism that would control fraud and waste.

In France and in the UK, the health care system pretty much covers everyone, but how are services paid? In the UK, they are paid by a tax for health care. This tax is about 12% for the individual and 13% for corporations. In France, the individuals pay about 9% and corporations pay 13%. The poor don't pay; however, the rich do pay. Statutory health insurance (the scheme in France) is financed by employer and employee payroll taxes (50%); a national earmarked income tax (35%); taxes levied on tobacco and alcohol, the pharmaceutical industry, and voluntary health insurance companies (13%); and state subsidies (2%). The taxes are not capped based on income. In some countries, prescriptions, dentistry, and optometry are not covered, so they are covered with private insurances. What is common is that there is a method that all countries use to mitigate risk and control costs. Mostly, this is done by limiting the services and/or products that are covered. What is not covered by the country is mostly covered by the insurance companies.

Theirs vs. Ours

Previously, we looked at a chart of the health care expenditures around the world. This chart tells us what health care costs in each country.

Health Care Expenditures Percent of GDP	as	Per-capita Spending ($USD)	Public Expenditure on Health, Percent of Total
Belgium	11.0%	$3,995	27.9%
Brazil	8.4%	$606	79.9%
Canada	10.4%	$4,079	70.2%
China	4.7%	$108	67.9%
France	11.4%	$3,696	77.8%
Germany	10.9%	$3,737	76.8%
Luxembourg	6.8%	$4,237	84.1%
Mexico	6.4%	$852	46.9%
Portugal	10%	$2,108	70.6%
Switzerland	11.2%	$4,627	59.1%
UK	10.1%	$3,129	82.6%
United States	17.6%	$8,086	46.5%

The first thing that is seen is in most of the countries represented on the chart, the percentage of GDP that is spent on health care is about 10%, and the cost per capita is about $4,000. But the thing that really sticks out is that the United States spends about double per capita for health care, and it consumes about 70% more of the percentage of GDP. The other thing that can be deemed from this chart is that the government in the United States only pays 46.5% of the cost of health care. The only country in this chart whose government pays less is Belgium. Belgium was ranked about twentieth in the world in 2000 according to the WHO. In other words, their government spends less on health care than in the United States, and the system is better.

There are things that this chart doesn't say. The public expenditure on health just measures the cost to the government, and not to the people. Yes, in the chart it does say per capita, and it gives you the amount that is spent per person. But that doesn't tell the whole story. It is easy to take the total cost of health care and divide it by the people in the country. That tells a story, but the real story is in the number of people who pay into the system and those who do not pay. When you start looking at how much those who pay actually pay, the story is different. Some people in other countries pay five times the cost per capita, and some pay more. Then those people must pay for health insurance also. It was stated earlier that most countries in the world have a mix between the government paying and a private insurance company paying what is left over. The chart states that most countries pay between 70% and 80% of total health expenditures. That is because private insurance companies pick up where the government left off.

In the United States, the insurance companies use pooling to lower the cost of insurance on average. This is done by risk to the pool. Those who are sick or unhealthy will pay more, and those who are healthy will pay less. That makes the average to the pool less and allows for a profit for the insurance company. In other countries, the pool is based on income, who can afford to pay and how much. The Fraser Institute in Canada did a study and found that the cost of health care ranges from about $500 per year for the poor to about $59,000 per year for those in the highest tax bracket. In the UK, for example, if you have income of £100,000, you will pay £12,000. If you make £9,100, you will pay about £1,100. The question is, If the average cost of health care in the UK is about £3,200 per year or $4,000 in Canada, how many times should a person with a high income pay for health care?

In almost every system, there is a cost to the people. In the United States, before the ACA, private insurance cost the people about $5,900 per year. Medicare was paid by contributions from payroll taxes over many years (this is the way it is supposed to be run), and Medicaid was free to those on the system. In other words, the poor doesn't pay, and those who have insurance and Medicare pay. The average cost to the average person with health insurance was about 8.4% of earnings ($6,700/$80,000) in 2017. Remember that the average person also has to pay 1.45% for Medicare, and a percentage of their income tax goes to pay for Medicaid.

France has a tax on the people of 9%, and the people also must pay for insurance. The big difference is that in the United States, you don't pay for health insurance based on earnings. You pay based on your health risk to the insurance company. This means that in France, a person can be healthy and young and still pay 9% for insurance. This becomes a problem when the person starts making the equivalent of more than $100,000. Imagine paying $18,000 or $50,000 for health insurance because you make a bunch of money. In the United States, things are different.

Why does health care cost twice as much for health care in the United States as it does in Europe? There can be several answers from limitations in chronic coverage to smaller population size. At least 40% of the difference can be attributed to the difference in the cost of living. Maybe the difference in cost can be that every country has a different mechanism to manage risk. Managing risk is one reason. The biggest problem that the United States has is fraud and waste. The next largest cost is administration. Following administration is the uninsured. The uninsured cost is about 5% of the budgets for hospitals.

The biggest advantage that the countries with universal health care have over the United States is that, for the most part, they can limit fraud, waste, and payment risk. Because in most cases there is no payment risk and no fraud and waste, the cost of the system is necessarily lower.

In all the systems, the two things that must be addressed are risk and cost. This is what drives every business and every government. In most countries, the way that risk is addressed is by limiting the illnesses that are covered or the number of times that a person can have an illness like drug addiction. The cost component is generally not addressed or is addressed by price fixing. Some countries, like Canada, negotiate prices for drugs with the pharmaceutical companies and subsidize the cost.

In the United States, the question of risk and cost is not addressed effectively in the government programs. To drive this point home, Medicaid is essentially a point of service program that serves the poor. There is no risk to the people covered; all the risk and all the cost is incurred by the government. This cost is passed to the taxpayers. The only ways that Medicaid mitigates risk is to predetermine payments for procedures and to mandate approval for some procedures and drugs. In this system, there is waste and fraud that account for between $75 billion and $150 billion (GAO estimates). The cost of the program is about $580 billion with costs split between state and federal governments.

Before the expansion of Medicaid by the ACA, there were about 55 million people on Medicaid. Now there are about 76 million. It costs about $7,600 per person per year. If you extrapolated that number out to cover everyone in the United States, it would cost about $2.5 trillion per year, increasing yearly faster than inflation. The problem with Medicaid is not the $2.5 trillion, but how it is paid. Medicaid is paid with tax dollars, income tax dollars, from the states and the federal government. Imagine what would happen if everyone were on Medicaid and it was administered the same as it is now. That would mean that the states would be on the hook for about $1 trillion, and the federal government would pay about $1.5 trillion. You would go to the store and pay $5 for a loaf of bread, and the sales tax would be $2. But if you look really hard, you will see a benefit. To cover everyone, it would only cost $2.5 trillion. That is an improvement over the $2.7 trillion that we were paying before the ACA or the $3.3 trillion that we are paying today.

Medicare and Medicaid Advantages and Disadvantages

By analyzing Medicaid, there are a few things that need to be included in the perfect system. First, Medicaid is close to a point of service system that could allow anyone on the plan to get service and not have to pay, just present a card. Second, Medicaid picks up where Medicare leaves off. It pays for long-term care, chronic ailments, and covers the poor. Finally, Medicaid has a payment schedule. Ease of use and coverage of every ailment should be taken from Medicaid to include in the new system. Canada has a system that is close to Medicaid.

Medicare is also util. It allows those over sixty-five to have coverage without paying a huge amount to insurance companies. The coverage is basically point of service, and it operates very similar to the universal health care services around the world. It is interesting to note that a real "Medicare for all" is what most of the world has in place. The government picks up 70 or 80% of the cost of health care, and the rest is covered by private insurance that is paid by the individual.

We already know that the Medicaid system is great from a service point of view, but it is not great when it comes to cost. Medicare is about the same as Medicaid when it comes to cost. But we have a system in the United States that is about 50% cheaper than Medicare: private insurance. Prior to the ACA, it cost about $5,900 per person per year for insurance companies to provide insurance for their customers, and they still make a 4–5% profit or about $300 per person per year.

Building a Plan

How is it done? How can a plan be built that eliminates fraud and waste, has a util payment mechanism and serves all the people for the lowest cost? The way to handle the big questions is not to address them at all. Build a basic plan that covers the basics. The problem that the United States has is that we try to address every problem and devise systems that are built for the needs of the few, and not the needs of the many. There is a big reason that health care costs so much. It is not because of fraud and waste or administrative costs. That is almost 50% of the cost of the systems we have in place now. The real problem is that we keep designing systems that are based on the needs of a few people. Medicare is designed for the old, Medicaid is for the poor, and the ACA was built for those who still were excluded. The issue is the 1% of the people in the United States spends $90,000 or more on health care per year. That means that 1% of the population spends about $300,000,000,000, and we design systems for this rather than focusing on the $3 trillion that the other 99% spend.

The key in building a plan that will address the 99% and still meet the needs of the 1% is not to build for huge expenses but for small expenses and let economics take care of the big things. In other words, build a basic plan that everyone gets and a catastrophic insurance plan that would catch the needs of that 1% with huge expenses. The beauty is that when you start at the bottom and build up, sometimes the big issues tend to go away. In systems with a profit motive, fraud and waste tend to go away, so the government can't run this system.

The system also has to have competition to naturally drive down prices. The biggest part of this system is to eliminate extra taxes on any of the components of the system. The special taxes on insurance companies and the suchlike imposed by the ACA would disappear.

The basic plan would include a doctor's visit every six months, a physical with blood work the first $500 of prescriptions per year. Everything above that in a year goes against a lifetime cap of $1 million. In a nutshell, everyone has a lifetime cap, but they can use it to get any care they need or perceive that they need. The lifetime cap will be indexed to the CPI.

What about the people who need more than $1 million in coverage? What if you have to go to the doctor more than two times a year? The people who need more than $1 million in coverage can buy more coverage. If you must use care, the care will be available at all times. It just goes against your lifetime cap.

The truth is very few people use more than $1 million of health care in a lifetime. The first million is costly because people use coverage up to this amount. Over $1 million, there are much fewer people who use it. Over $2 million, there is an even smaller amount of people who use this level of services. The truth is most people die of what they have before they hit the first million or two. This is how supply and demand works. If a person knows that they don't have two or three chronic illnesses, they most likely don't have to buy two or three million dollars in coverage.

Notice that the 1% will be those purchasing the coverage above $1 million. The additional coverage will be inexpensive. "During one's lifetime, over $400K will be spent on the average American's healthcare in today's dollars. And that is if medical costs rise as the same rate as inflation. If medical costs rise at 3% more than inflation, your healthcare will cost over $2MM, the vast majority of which will take place after the age of 45" (https://www.registerednursing.org/healthcare-costs-by-age/).

Looking at the big questions, birth control, fertility treatment, etc., I think they can go against the lifetime cap. Abortion will not be covered. That doesn't mean that a person cannot obtain an abortion. They just must pay for it out of pocket. Birth control pills are prescriptions, so it is covered in the basic plan.

By setting a basic plan, the costs per unit of time can be projected. As an example, two doctor's visits at $150 per visit and basic blood work $300 plus $500 in prescription drugs are equal to $1,100 for the year. Second, by setting a lifetime cap, the payer will be able to project the capital requirements that need to be met based on how many people use each level of coverage. Finally, by using this methodology, it will not just control waste, fraud, risk, and cost, but it will also empower the covered to make medical/health decisions without being encumbered by the government or insurance companies. The individual would have control over his/her own health care account to manage in any fashion they deem fit.

In essence, this plan is composed of a predictable basic plan and a capped "catastrophic" insurance plan. The catastrophic plan can be easily priced across the entire population to determine the simple cost of the complete plan. The cost of the first part of the plan can be about $1,100, and the cost of the second part of the plan can be about $2,400. The total cost of the entire plan should be about $3,500 per person per year. The aggregate cost on health care in this plan would be about $1.155 trillion per year ($3,500 x 330 million people). Clearly, this is not the total cost for health care, just this part of the plan.

The beauty of the plan is that costs can be determined, and because the government and the insurance companies have no stake in the outcome or payment, the individual has control over spending and services. The purpose of a cap on spending is twofold: first, to determine the risk to the payer, and second, once the risk is determined, the payer will have no interest in what is spent. The liability is constrained.

Now that we have this big plan with everyone on it, how do we pay for it? The UK has a point-of-service system that is paid for by a special tax. Canada has a tax to pay for health care. However, Germany is the inspiration for a payment mechanism. It is a multipayer system that is paid for by way of a payroll tax of about 15% split between the people and their employers. There is a rationale for using the payroll tax as a payment mechanism. The payroll tax is a simple choice. It is the way that almost every country uses for its people to pay for their health care.

Currently, the average person pays three times for health care. The goal of this scheme is for the average person only to pay once for health care. That means no portion of income taxes should go to health care, just the payroll tax.

New Health Care Plan

The biggest problem with designing a health care system is focus. Most of the schemes both in the United States and around the world focus on fixing things for a small amount of people that may cost a tremendous amount and applying this system to everyone. This makes the scheme expensive. Medicare is focused on serving a growing portion of the country that accounts for about one-fourth of the population but, at any given time, may have exorbitant expenditures. Medicaid covers about the same amount of people as Medicare; however, it may contain some people who are chronically ill. The ACA covers less than 10% of the people in the country, but a large percentage of those people would be considered adversely selected by insurance companies. The fact is that more than 50% of the people in the United States spend less than $250 per year in health care. Rather than focus on the anomalies, any health care scheme needs to focus on the majority of people and build in systems for those chronically ill or elderly.

Quite simply put, there are two main parts to health care: the service itself and the payment mechanism. In the United States, the problem is not in the health care service. It is expensive compared to the rest of the world, but the problem is in the payment mechanism. A great number of people do not have access to health care because of the cost. That is why a new system must be easy to pay for from a government standpoint and from the standpoint of the people who will be paying.

Currently, some people pay multiple times to get one plan. That is, if a person has an employer-sponsored plan, they may pay what the company doesn't pay. Then the person still must pay the Medicare part of payroll tax. Then there is a component of income tax that goes to pay for Medicaid.

A new health care plan must simplify the payments for the people and standardize a plan or group of plans that will allow 100% of the people to control their health care and pay once.

The most important part of this plan is to simplify how health care will be paid for and make it available for everyone without deductibles or copayments.

Here is a summary of the plan outlining one of the options and the general layout of how the overall plan will function. This plan will use what is already in place for implementation and administration. The plan will be less expensive, and everyone in the country will be covered. This plan will show how to cover 100% of the population of the United States without raising federal income taxes, destroying the pharmaceutical industry, the medical industry, or health insurance industry. The plan will keep in place competition that will drive down costs. It will shift responsibility from the government to the private sector and eliminate Medicare and Medicaid.

The first step is to build a basic plan that covers the basics: a doctor's visit every six months, a physical with blood work, and the first $500 of prescriptions per year. Everything above that in a year goes against a lifetime cap of $1 million. What is fashioned is a basic plan with a defined cost and a secondary component that is a catastrophic insurance plan that pays for anything outside the basic plan.

In a nutshell, everyone has a lifetime cap, but they can use it to get any care they need or perceive that they need. The lifetime cap will be indexed to the CPI. A few of the big questions that will come up are, "What about the people who need more than $1 million in coverage?" "What if you have to go to the doctor more than two times a year?"

There are simple answers. The people who need more than $1 million in coverage can buy more coverage. If you must use care, the care will be available at all times. It just goes against your lifetime cap. The truth is very few people use more than $1 million of health care in a lifetime. The first million is costly because people use coverage up to this amount. Over $1 million, there are much fewer people who use it. Over $2 million, there is an even smaller amount of people who use this level of services. The truth is most people die of what they have before they hit the first million or two. Abortion will not be covered. That doesn't mean that a person cannot obtain an abortion, they just must pay for it out of pocket. Birth Control pills are prescriptions so it is covered in the basic plan.

In any plan there must be a way to project cost on a yearly basis, even a monthly basis for the payer. If the plan is similar to the ACA or Medicare for all and mandates coverage for pregnancy, e.g., medication, cancer treatments, etc., then there is no definition, no way to predict what the payer will have to pay in any unit of time, except to use statistics.

By setting a basic plan, the costs per unit of time can be projected. As an example, two doctor's visits at $150 per visit and basic blood work $300 plus $500 in prescription drugs are equal to $1,100 for the year. Second, by setting a lifetime cap, the payer will be able to project the capital requirements that need to be met based on how many people use each level of coverage. Finally, by using this methodology, it will not just control waste, fraud, risk, and cost, but it will also empower the covered to make medical/health decisions without being encumbered by the government or insurance companies. The individual would have control over his/her own health care account to manage in any fashion they deem fit.

In essence, this plan is composed of a predictable basic plan and a capped "catastrophic" insurance plan. The catastrophic plan can be easily priced across the entire population to determine the simple cost of the complete plan. The cost of the first part of the plan can be about $1,100, and the cost of the second part of the plan can be about $2,400. The total cost of the entire plan should be about $3,500 per person per year. The aggregate cost on health care in this plan would be about $1.155 trillion per year ($3,500 x 330 million people). Clearly, this is not the total cost for health care, just this part of the plan.

The beauty of the plan is that costs can be determined, and because the government and the insurance companies have no stake in the outcome or payment, the individual has control over spending and services. The purpose of a cap on spending is twofold: first, to determine the risk to the payer, and second, once the risk is determined, the payer will have no interest in what is spent. The liability is constrained.

This is a quick outline that will show the simplicity of the plan:

1) Two-part plan: basic coverage and catastrophic plan
2) The government will contract with the insurance companies through a fixed-price contract to administer and make payments for the plan.
3) People will pay 10% of salary or wages over $35,000, 5% of salary or wages under $25,000 for health care. Between $25,000

and \$35,000, the rate will rise from 5%–10%. This will be paid directly into the payroll tax for Medicare. Medicare recipients will pay \$100 per month.

4) The states will continue to pay Medicaid payments. These payments will be \$3,500 for every citizen in the state who makes less than \$25,000. This includes children.

5) Employers will contribute \$100 per employee per month or 7% of wages, whichever is smaller, through the payroll tax

6) Everyone will be on a standard plan that encourages preventative care. There should be a lifetime cap of \$1 million. Everything above the standard plan on a yearly basis goes against the lifetime cap. There are other options that allow for higher caps or different services.

7) Everything is covered (except cosmetic procedures and abortion), no copay, no deductibles.

8) The first \$500 per year of prescriptions are covered. Everything else goes against the lifetime cap. This \$500 is a placeholder. It is a mechanism that allows a person to opt for dental care, vision care, or any number of services that are normal to health care.

FRAMEWORK

Insurance Companies

The most important part of this plan is the insurance companies. The insurance companies will act as the payment mechanism and administration for the plan. There will be a minimum plan. The basic plan will have a lifetime maximum benefit of $1 million in which most will opt. The insurance companies will be allowed to sell policies that are similar to this plan with altered goals. The argument against lifetime maximums is that some people need more coverage. The benefit here is we allow the insurance companies to lower risk and sell additional coverage at prices that are extremely low.

Insurance companies already have networks in place, so rolling over into a new system would be as simple as tying a shoe. There is a benefit to capping the insurance companies upper limit. Because the function of the insurance companies is to administer the system and make payments with their risks capped, they have no interest in what a person does with their money. This will allow the person or the individual to make all treatment decisions. This benefit also creates a cottage industry in consulting with patients who need assistance in making medical decisions. This void can be filled by the government, the health care providers, or private industry.

In essence, insurance companies will enter into a contract with the federal government for a fixed payment per person that they cover. Their goal is to cover as many people as possible. This creates competition between the insurance companies and will result in added benefits that could include greater services like gym memberships and bonuses for not smoking. The insurance companies will submit the people whom they cover to the government, and the government will pay the insurance companies directly on a per person basis. This will be a fixed contract. It is the insurance company's job to make a profit.

Government

The government will pool the taxes collected from the workforce and pay the insurance companies on a per person basis. It will be a fixed-price contract with every insurance company. The current Medicare part of the payroll tax will be the mechanism to collect taxes used to pay the insurance companies. Medicare and Medicaid will be annexed, saving the federal government $800 billion per year. The major function for the government in this plan will be to police the plan so there is no corruption.

Because of the need for counseling for patients who may not be able to make medical decisions, there is an opportunity for the government to provide this type of assistance. It can be a free service, or the government can opt to contract with other companies to aid people with medical decisions.

The most important part of this plan is that it pays for itself. The revenues that are raised are used to pay for the health care of all the people. The tax rates and other revenue generation will pay for the total cost of the plan. The accounting for this plan can look like $1.155 trillion in expenses and $1.155 trillion in revenue. There will be no line item for income tax because this is a separate method of payment. Furthermore, there are no subsidies for this program, no cost to income tax.

The Individual

Every individual will use their Social Security number or Green Card to register with the insurance company of their choice to participate in the plan. Everyone in the workforce will pay 10% of their wages or salary in payroll tax to pay for the plan. The 10% will be capped at a salary of $150k (this can be tweaked to raise or lower revenue). Those who make less than $25,000 will pay 5% of their wages for the plan. Between $25,000 and $35,000, the tax will increase gradually from 5% to 10%.

Those currently enrolled in Medicare will be absorbed into the plan and pay $100 per month. This tax will be collected through the current Social Security mechanism. The individual will have an option of how to use the plan that addresses the needs of that individual. People who are on unemployment will pay 5% out of their unemployment check for the insurance. Those who cannot work will be paid for by Social Security Disability. The homeless and those not working and/or not in the workforce will be paid for by the state in which they reside. Those on government social programs will have an aggregate amount of 5% reduced from their benefits to pay for the health care plan. The goal is to incentivize work.

Corporations

Companies will pay $100 per employee per month or 7% of the employee's wage, whichever is less. This tax will be collected through the current Medicare mechanism of payroll taxes. The individual's 1099 and contract labor will be responsible to pay for their coverage through the self-employment tax. This is different than in other countries in the world because in general the burden on companies is generally a straight percentage. Setting a fixed cost will allow companies to plan to hire and compensate. No longer will companies have to provide health care as a benefit. Companies will be responsible for providing a mechanism for employees to sign up for health care.

State Governments

This is one of the keys to the plan. Since we will be absorbing Medicaid, we will need the states to continue to pay into the system the equivalent amount that they are paying for Medicaid. Furthermore, the states will need to pick up some of the slack of children, homeless, and the people who are not employed and have no support. This number is a fixed amount. The states will pay $3,500 per year for every person in the individual state who is not working or is a child under eighteen.

THE MATH

The math is basic. When you add the average cost of the basic services, including the cost of prescriptions, the cost per person per year is about $1,100 or about $363 billion. That is the first component of the cost of the system. The second part of the cost is the amount to cover the $1,000,000 of insurance and the profit for the insurance companies. This is the hard part. Without going into actuarial tables, we can estimate that the insurance part of this equation will be about $792 billion. Simplified, the cost can be about $200 per person per month. Without going into specifics, the number was derived by taking the present value of lifetime payments to total an average cost of a lifetime benefit.

Revenue Side

The total cost of health care in the new system should be about $1.155 trillion. As mentioned earlier, current Medicare enrollees will be absorbed into the plan and will contribute about $120 per month per person or about $93.6 billion. The unemployed with contribute $7.2 billion. The Medicaid contribution from the states should be about $245 billion. The contribution from the workforce will be about $814.7 trillion. The total amount of revenue is about $1.161 trillion

The breakdown of workforce and corporate contributions is as follows (numbers are rounded):

Breakdown of Workforce and Corporate Contributions				
Income Level	Number of People in Level	Individual Contribution	Corporate Contribution	Total Yearly Contribution
Under $25k	75 million	$1000	$1000	$150 billion
$25k - $50k	42 million	$4600	$1200	$243.6 billion
$50k – $75	25 million	$6700	$1200	$197.5 billion
$75k - $100k	8 million	$9000	$1200	$81.6 billion
$100k +	10 million	$13000	$1200	$142 billion

The Other Side of the Equation

The math shows how the funds for the pool are going to be collected. The other side of the equation is what the government pays the insurance companies to administer the plan. This is easily defined as the total cost of health care, $1.155 trillion divided by the total amount of citizens, 330 million. The government pays the insurance companies about $3,500 per person per year.

The way it will work is the government will collect the pool of taxes, and every month, insurance companies will present their list of enrollees to the government, and the government will pay them. The insurance companies are responsible for all payments to health care providers. People will be able to utilize any health care service at any time without worry or cost (other than the payroll tax). Everyone born will get a Social Security card and be enrolled in this plan. The clock starts to tick on the lifetime benefit at birth. Everyone with a Social Security card or Green Card will be included. Others will not.

The plan will be a contract between the government and all insurance companies in the country. There should be a law that states that the taxes collected for this contract cannot be diverted for any other purpose, and any bill proposed to divert funds from this pool is punishable by a prison term.

COMMENTS AND ADDITIONAL INFORMATION

As you can see, the plan is quite simple. Any increases to the workforce as a percentage of citizens will lower the cost per person working. As health care costs increase, there will be a corresponding increase in payment to insurance companies indexed to the CPI. There is also a huge downside risk. If the workforce shrinks or decreases, the burden of the payments shifts. This would leave the government to make up the cost of the difference to fund the health care plan or to build in a rainy-day fund.

Interestingly enough, the cost of care to cover the entire country will decrease to a level similar to that of the rest of the industrial world with single-payer systems. The huge difference between this plan and the Patient Protection and Affordable Care Act is one shifts the cost to the private sector and the other keeps the cost in the public sector.

There is another incidental effect of this system. Because everyone will be covered by the program, there is no payment risk. This is extremely important because one of the reasons that hospitals charge a lot for an aspirin or a box of tissues is the payment risk that they incur because of the uninsured. The flip side of this equation is that there are more people that will exercise choice, there will be more competition, and the price of services should decrease.

One-Million-Dollar Cap

It is important to cap the lifetime benefits. Unlimited benefits lead to greater risk for insurance companies, which mean higher costs. The incidental effect is that insurance companies will not be making health care decisions; the individual will make all choices based on the amount of coverage available. No death panels. This also allows people to explore experimental treatments without interference from insurance companies, the government, or outside sources.

Corporations

Corporations should embrace this system. Those who provide health care have a set figure to pay to provide health care. Those companies who don't provide health care can adjust costs to include health care costs as a fixed cost. Most companies that provide health insurance will embrace this system because it will actually decrease the cost of providing health insurance for them.

Insurance Companies

Insurance companies will love this system. They increase their risk pool, including young healthy people who are not currently covered, the payments are guaranteed, and the profit is almost built in. There is opportunity for growth because many people will opt to buy other types of insurance and higher dollar amounts in excess of $1 million.

There is another benefit for the insurance companies. When the computations for the lifetime benefits were done, they were based on the future value of $2,400 per year for forty years to arrive at $400,000, the average amount that the average person will spend in health care for their lifetime. The great benefit for insurance companies is that the premiums are not just paid for forty years, but for the lifetime of the person, which now can be eighty years.

Individuals

This is the easy part of the equation. Every individual will be able to choose his insurance company and the level of coverage. Every condition is covered, and experimental drugs are covered. There are no copays and no deductibles. The decision-making process for treatment is determined by the individual and his doctor. Cost is determined by salary, and most will either lower payment or go from no insurance to having insurance.

The Government

The problem is that the government will save billions per year with this system. The new system will put thousands of government employees out of work and cut government spending.

It has been said that the reason that there is no change in the government is because too many people are dependent on the current government programs to make a living. It is not about making things better. It is about making additional programs that support a current program so that political donors can be paid.

There is a built-in counseling component of this plan for people who cannot make informed health care decisions. This will allow the government to contract to outside companies who can provide this service or give assistance to those who are signing up for the program. This way, the government will be able to add an additional program and spend the taxpayer's money.

RATIONALE

There are a few other issues that need to be covered. There are several options to the basic plan. Part of the basic plan is $500 per year in prescription drugs. This is a placeholder for a couple of options. Not all people need prescription drugs, so this $500 can be used for eye care and/or dental care. The amount can also be used for a combination of prescriptions, eye and dental, or any combination of the three.

The most important part of the new plan is that the catastrophic coverage can be expanded. The average person will spend $400,000 in his/her lifetime; however, many people will spend multiples of that amount. That is the reason that some people need to purchase more than $1 million in coverage. The beauty of the structure of the new plan is that the second million is cheaper than the first and the third million is cheaper than the second.

One thing that needs to be stressed is that fact that the new plan is defined. That means that the cost of the plan can be determined for the most part. The basic part of the plan in every region can be determined by the average cost of a doctor's visit, the cost of medical tests, and the $500 for extras. The catastrophic insurance plan can be determined by figuring the cost of the plan across the population and taking the average. There are no other parts to the plan. Insurance companies can sell the second, third, and fourth million in coverage to derive a larger profit, or this can be given to derive a competitive edge. On the other side of the equation, the government can add their cost to collect the funds, make payments, and police the plan to the cost of the plan to the individual.

The new plan must comply with economics. Because there will be more demand for health care and the supply in the short run will be the same, the prices for health care services will be higher. This can be offset by competition. There will be no price fixing. This will stop shortages. No products or services should be sold below cost by the government to offset high prices.

Subsidies

One of the biggest issues is that those making less than $25,000 may be able to pay for a couple of doctor's visits and perhaps some prescriptions, but there is no way that they would be able to afford a full-blown insurance plan without subsidies.

Subsidies is an issue that needs to be addressed. The government estimates that it will spend $1.039 trillion on subsidies for the ACA in the period from 2015 and 2024 (https://www.thebalance.com/government-subsidies-definition-farm-oil-export-etc-3305788). That is an average of about $100 billion per year. When the new plan was developed, one of the things that was crucial was to avoid subsidies and government transfer payments to anyone. This practice makes any scheme costlier to those who are actually paying. As discussed previously, in other countries, those earning lower than a predetermined income are not required to pay for services and receive them for free. This adds to the burden that those who pay have to pay. It is for that reason that everybody pays something—everyone has skin in the game.

A simple rationale is that if there are a hundred people paying for something that a hundred people are receiving, then the cost per person is lowered. On the other side of the equation, if thirty people are paying for a hundred people to have a service that fifty get for free and twenty get subsidized, the cost to those thirty people is going to be multiple times the amount paid by those receiving a subsidy. Furthermore, to generate the subsidy, the government would have to levee a higher tax on those paying taxes to support the system.

It is for this reason that the decision was made that everyone will pay. Everyone pays for Medicare that they may or may not receive at the age of sixty-five so there will be a payment required from everyone in this system.

COUNSELING

Because of the nature of the new plan, there will be a lot of people who will need help with how to manage their accounts and health care decisions. The issue is that since the government is no longer making any financial decisions for the people and the insurance companies have a maximum that they have to pay out, there is no interest in the individual accounts. The individual is in charge of their own health care, their own decisions. For those who cannot manage their accounts, there needs to be a mechanism that will aid people with decisions financially and health-wise.

Preexisting conditions

There are several people who will have a need for more than the $1 million plan. Those people will need to purchase more coverage. As mentioned, the new plan is built for the masses and not the 1% who spend more than $90,000 per year in health care. So those who have chronic illnesses, alcoholism, drug addiction, and those who smoke will have to buy additional coverage. This is another beauty of the new plan. Because the first level of catastrophic insurance covers $1 million and 99% of the people will not use this level of service, the 1% who have to purchase more than $1 million in coverage will not have to pay huge amounts for additional coverage. Those with preexisting conditions will not be excluded.

Lightning Source UK Ltd.
Milton Keynes UK
UKHW010224021020
370885UK00002B/43/J

9 781664 123984